T'AI CHI
IN A CHAIR

FAIR WINDS
PRESS

GLOUCESTER, MASSACHUSETTS

First published in the USA in 2001 by
Fair Winds Press
33 Commercial Street
Gloucester, MA 01930

10 9 8 7 6 5 4 3 2 1

Printed and bound in Canada

Cover design by Jane Ramsey
Book design by Faith Hague
Illustrations by Jane Ramsey

ISBN 1-931412-60-X

*The information in this book is for educational purposes only.
It is not intended to replace the advice of a physician or medical
practitioner. Please see your health care provider before beginning
any new health program.*

Contents

To my mother, Mary; my husband, Rick;
my daughter, Michelle; and my son-in-law, Ian
for their love and support.

Acknowledgments

I would like to express my deepest gratitude to my family, friends, teachers, and students whose encouragement, support, and help have made this book possible. My particular thanks go out to the residents of Cambridge Court who offered themselves as research subjects in the formation of this exercise system especially to Kathleen Holm, Roman Fink, Peggy Jorgensen, Rita O'Rourke, Betty Arneson, Irene Larson, Onetta Schaefer, Cliff Weir, Wanda Stenberg, Jean Goodman, Renae Lynch, and my friend Ruth Ross, now deceased.

To my students at the Senior Citizens' Center: Mary Ann Komar, Vera Huston, Mae Caufield, Evelyn McKenna, Don and Jean Bartsch , and Mary Louise Anderson.

To my instructors: Pat Moore and Jan Marcus.

To massage therapists: Annette Welsh, Mike Dalton and Una Koontz for introducing me to the health benefits of massage and for their instructions in the use and value of acupressure points.

To Donald G. Hollenhorst for setting me on a life-long path of excitement and discovery in the field of philosophy.

To my editor at Fair Winds Press, Holly Schmidt, for her patience, advice, and encouragement.

To Jane Ramsey, for her wonderful illustrations of the exercises in this book.

Introduction

Within the pages of this book is a comprehensive wellness program based on the Yang style of T'ai Chi Chu'an along with an easy-to-understand guide to the healing benefits of acupressure and self-massage. You may choose to use Chapter 3, which comprises the hour-long seated exercises, or you may prefer to practice the fifteen-minute daily exercise routines that contain a list of helpful acupressure points to enhance the healing quality of each day's exercises, as described in Chapter 4. No matter which routine you select, the soft, flowing, painless movements of seated T'ai Chi will help you to achieve your ideal weight by stimulating your natural energy. This energy will flow to and through your body's organs and systems while your bones, muscles, and joints are being exercised and strengthened. In addition, Chapter 5 provides directions for locating acupressure points that will speed recovery and alleviate pain for anything from a toothache to a broken bone. Regardless of your age, gender, or level of physical fitness—without ever leaving your living room—this seated T'ai Chi progam will increase your energy, optimize your feeling of well-being, and bring your "self" into harmony with your surroundings.

How Seated T'ai Chi Began

"One who thinks everything is easy
inevitably finds everything difficult.
That is why the Sage alone
regards everything as difficult
and in the end
finds no difficulty at all."

—*LAO TZU (CH. 63)*

When I first began my job as the program supervisor at a retirement community, I had been studying dance and martial arts for many years. This experience led me to develop a program of dance and martial arts–based exercises for the senior citizens who participated in my exercise classes. At that time, all of the residents were independent retirees who required little or no assistance with their daily activities. When the facility changed from one for independent seniors to an assisted-living community, I had to reevaluate the entire activities program.

While many of the standard activities were age and condition appropriate, the exercise classes had to be altered dramatically to target the growing number of residents who were dependent on walkers, canes, or wheelchairs.

My challenge was to find exercises that accommodated all of the participants, those able to stand for a limited period of time and those unable to stand at all. In addition, this new program had to be designed in such a way that the purpose of any exercise program (i.e., strengthening, flexibility, improved circulation, fat burning, etc.) was not lost through over modification. The result was a seated exercise program based on traditional movements found in the Yang style of T'ai Chi Chu'an. What I found was that this program resulted in a dramatic change in the health and fitness level of the participants. No matter what your age or your fitness level, seated T'ai Chi can do the same for you!

Eastern vs. Western Exercise Systems

Most Western exercise depends upon the number of repetitions and the rate of speed of each exercise for its efficacy. Robert Chuckrow, in *The Tai Chi Book*, compares our Western exercise systems to "trying to drive with the brakes on." We spend much of our time contracting muscles and, in the process, unconsciously pit one muscle group against another. The exercises become exhausting rather than energizing, painful and injurious rather than pleasant and healing. This is why people have difficulty sticking to a traditional exercise program. T'ai Chi, on the other hand, is a relaxed process with slow and meditative movements performed while the mind remains always alert to the spatial relationship between the body and its surroundings. Awareness of the air displaced by each movement and the symbiosis between one part of the body and another, for example, underscores the differences in approach between Western exercise and that found in Eastern countries. In addition, all T'ai Chi movements are performed with particular attention to a natural, but synchronized, pattern of breathing.

The importance placed on proper breathing by Asian cultures cannot be overstated. We in the West, particularly those of us not involved in the health field, view breathing as an involuntary act of the body, a responsibility assumed by the respiratory system without need for conscious intervention on our part. Conversely, in Japan and China, breathing exercises are prescribed for any number of medical conditions. These exercises range from a meditative process with little or no movement of the body (similar to that found in the Dragon's Breath exercise) to powerful exhalations produced by bending the body abruptly from the waist. The average citizen of these countries is just as apt to be given a prescription for a breathing workout as an herbal remedy or a trip to the acupuncturist.

Because it is the *mind* that controls the activity of the *ch'i* and the flow of its sparks of energy throughout the body, there is no need to do one hundred jumping jacks or run a 12-mile race to be in good shape The end result is the same as our standard Western exercises in terms of revitalizing muscles, bones, joints, and organs and increasing the flow of oxygen throughout the system. Furthermore, what better exercise could there be for the mind than that required in the practice of T'ai Chi? We must juggle several things at the same time. We must be cognizant of the area we have targeted, aware of the movement of energy, knowledgeable about the existence and location of meridians and their juncture points, concerned with the spatial relation between ourselves and our surroundings. The results are manifest. We rediscover our intimate connection to nature, our inherent physical strength, reawaken our intuitive abilities, expand our mental capacity, and develop our spiritual consciousness, all without a single stress fracture.

T'ai Chi Chu'an Forms

There are five styles of T'ai Chi Chu'an practiced today all over the world. They originated within certain families and therefore bear their names: Sun, Fu, Wu, Chen, and Yang. Paul Crompton, in *The T'ai Chi Workbook*, tells us that in addition to these five well-known styles, there are also an unknown number of "closed" family styles, which, as the term implies, are kept secret from all but members of the immediate family. While there is no consensus of opinion regarding the origin of T'ai Chi Chu'an itself, most practitioners seem to accept the Yang style as the basis of all other styles.

It would have been possible to simply take this very well-known Yang short form and redesign it for my elderly students to practice while seated. There is, however, the matter of the integrity of the form itself. Within any T'ai Chi form, there lies a certain inherent logic and purpose to each of the movements. The synchronization of the upper body with the steps and the breathing exists in a very carefully crafted order developed over hundreds of years. While simply transforming the Yang short style to a seated version would have made for an interesting exercise, it would not have served the purpose for which the form was originally intended. In addition, it was necessary to construct an exercise system that could be easily understood and performed by those with no experience in the martial arts and one that would concentrate our efforts on the particular areas of the body most in need of help.

Oddly enough, I found that, while these exercises were intended for my elderly students, I also benefited from them in ways that were totally unexpected. I felt that because I wasn't sweating and straining through a class that I would experience no improvement in my own condition. I have been amazed by the improvement in my breathing and the strengthening of the muscles of my arms and even my legs without the residual aches and pains associated with traditional aerobic exercise. My immune system seems to be working overtime and my stamina has increased tenfold. I no longer return home exhausted at the end of the day, nor have I suffered from the usual array of colds and flu that have been particularly plentiful this year.

T'ai Chi is not merely an exercise system for the body but, rooted as it is in Taoist philosophy, it is also a coming together of all facets of a human being—mind, body, and spirit. This truly holistic approach adds a new dimension to the concept of exercising and presented for me an even greater challenge to the development of an effective series of exercises that could be performed while sitting down. The result, which I believe to be a successful one, is the subject of this book.

T'ai Chi and the Taoist Philosophy

The secrecy surrounding the Chinese martial-arts systems have given rise to many legends regarding the establishment of the self defense/exercise system known as T'ai Chi Chu'an or grand ultimate fist. One school of thought attributes the origin of T'ai Chi to a fifteenth-century Taoist monk, Zhang San-feng, who witnessed a deadly battle between a crane and a snake. According to the story, Zhang believed the snake was victorious because of his relaxed, evasive movements and his lightning-fast counter strikes. Other practitioners of the art maintain that T'ai Chi Chu'an was not developed until somewhere around 1740. Whatever the true historical facts of its origins, T'ai

Chi has remained a dominant system of Kung Fu throughout China, and more recently, has become a popular form of exercise in the United States.

T'ai Chi is rooted in Taoist philosophy and based on the opposing principles of *yin* and *yang*, which, by their complementary nature, create harmony in the universe. T'ai Chi is, in fact, the physical expression of that philosophy, for traditional Chinese medicine teaches that illness is the result of the interruption of the flow of *ch'i* (life force) by the temporary imbalance of the body's forces. If one accepts the premise of Chinese medicine, then it stands to reason that all diseases can be cured by the rebalancing of the yin and yang and the return to free-flowing ch'i. An exercise system, therefore, that brings about or restores these two opposing forces to the proper balance would have the beneficial effect of returning the body to its normal healthful condition. That is the overall effect of T'ai Chi.

Yin and Yang

Chinese health practitioners view the human body as made up of meridians or pathways. These pathways connect organs, joints, and muscle groups to each other and to areas in which the skin can be pressed or punctured to relieve pain, release tension, and rebalance the particular parts of the body to which these spots on the skin are related. It is believed by some historians that there were originally anywhere from 365 to 500 pathways in use throughout the history of acupuncture. In this book, we will limit our use of acupressure points to the fourteen meridians, or pathways, as identified by Michael Reed Gach, in *Acupressure's Potent Points*: lung, large intestine, stomach, spleen, heart, small intestine, urinary bladder, kidney, pericardium, triple warmer, gallbladder, liver, and the Conception and Governing vessels. It is the processes of yin and yang that allow for the movement of ch'i through these meridians of the body.

The symbol used to represent yin and yang is a circle divided into two fish-shaped parts, one black and one white. The implication of the tiny circle of opposing color in each is, of course, that neither yin nor yang is wholly antithetical to the other.

Each of the two principles have both gender and quality designations. Yang is the male principle and that part of nature and man that is light, dry, active, strong, and hot. Yin is the female principle, encompassing that which is dark, wet, inactive, weak, and cold. These two elements are in a constant process of evolution, the one giving way to the other in an endless succession of dark to light, wet to dry, activity to rest, weakness into strength, and the heat of day into the coolness of night.

Yin and yang, while oppositional in their characteristics, are nevertheless not in conflict in their activities. As day follows night, so too does yin flow inevitably into yang. Some activities of these two principles as they seek a balance within the human body are unconscious, driven by the body's own regulating system. Others are the result of our conscious desire to be comfortable. During hot summer months, we seek a spot in the shade and a cool drink. All ranges of activity, then, whether consciously controlled or involuntary, are the function of yin and yang.

That which is regulated by the activities of yin and yang is ch'i. It is variously defined as life force, soul, spirit, or energy. When the word is used in the more universal sense, it is taken to mean the life force without which we would die. Within the context of this book, however, we will be using the word *ch'i* to mean the energy flowing through the meridians as we perform each exercise. Imagine, if you will, that ch'i is a vehicle traversing the pathways of our bodies. As long as these pathways remain clear and free of obstacles by virtue of the proper balance of yin and yang the ch'i can continue on its way. If, however, we have suffered an injury, have been ill, overindulged in the wrong kinds of foods, or neglected to exercise, then those pathways or meridians become blocked. Assuming that we do eat properly, get enough rest, and exercise regularly, all should be well.

More precisely still, and for the purpose of simplifying the visualizations that must accompany each exercise, we will imagine ch'i as a spinning disc residing in the lower abdomen. The *dan tien*, or spinning disc, is located in the center of the body, level with the area approximately three finger widths below the navel. With the opening exercises in the Breathing section, we set the disc in motion. As we breathe deeply and concentrate on ch'i, the disc spins faster and faster releasing showers of energy that travel wherever we direct them to go with our minds.

The Three Treasures

The ancient Chinese believed that those who develop the proper balance between mind, body, and breath are in possession of three treasures. Those treasures are named *jing*, *ch'i*, and *shen*. They can be found in three specific locations in the body called the *dan tiens*. The lower dan tien, which we discussed in the previous section, is believed to be the repository for jing, the middle dan tien for ch'i and the upper dan tien for shen. Jing refers to the energy or ch'i as it is expressed through movement away from the body such as that used against an opponent. The ch'i of the middle dan tien denotes the "breath" of the body, which is believed to reside in the middle dan tien in the area of the diaphragm, lungs, and solar plexus. Shen is related to all mental and spiritual activities.

Superficially, jing is identified with the sex organs, a man's sperm and testosterone, and a woman's ovaries and estrogen. Yet, the proper definition of this term includes the whole endocrine system and all of the chemical interactions of metabolism. Jing is our biochemical makeup; how we grow and develop, the strength or weakness of our constitution, how we age, and whether our body retains its youthful vigor or begins to deteriorate in middle age is determined by the quantity of jing available in the body. This is not necessarily, however, a preexisting condition but rather is dependent on the way in which we live our lives.

Ch'i that resides in the middle dan tien (located in the solar plexus) is most accurately defined as the functional energy of the body. Together with jing, it regulates maturation and aging. Ch'i is believed to be responsible for the involuntary functions of the body such as breathing and heartbeat as well as voluntary muscle activity. Ch'i also controls the circulation, particularly the amount of oxygen in the blood as well as the processes of the nervous system.

Shen is associated with mental activity. Decision making, academic achievements, analytical thought, and impulse control all fall within the purview of shen. When expanded through meditation and concentrated effort, *shen* takes on a higher aspect related to intuition, creativity, and spirituality. Because we concentrate our efforts and our minds on the three dan tiens in our T'ai Chi exercises, we will be activating the properties or treasures that reside in these locations.

The Three *Dan Tiens*

The three dan tiens that house the Three Treasures, are, therefore, the cultivation points from which all energy flows. The lower dan tien is thought to be located between the pubic bone and the navel about midway through the body. The lower dan tien is connected in Chinese medicine to the kidneys and is believed to be the source of a person's power, particularly when T'ai Chi is used as a *martial* art. The middle dan tien, as mentioned previously, is in the middle of the body in the area of the solar plexus and relates to general physical vitality. The upper dan tien is to be found in the area of the pineal gland. To measure its precise position, draw an imaginary line from the tops of your ears through your head and another line from between the eyebrows (the Third Eye Point) straight to the back of your head. Where the two horizontal lines intersect is the location of the upper dan tien.

The Eight Meridians

In order to be able to visualize the movement of energy through the body as we do in all the exercises described in this book, we need to know what routes we wish the energy to take.

That, in turn, depends on which part of the body we are targeting and what we hope to accomplish. The following is a list of the eight meridians:

1. The *dumei* begins at the perineum, rises up the back and along the center line of the body, over the scalp, down the forehead, ending at the upper palate of the mouth behind the teeth.
2. The *renmei* moves from the tip of the tongue, down the center line of the front of the body and back to the perineum.
3. The *chongmei* is a line that begins at the perineum and runs vertically through the three dan tien points.
4. The *daimei* resembles a belt encircling the waist that starts and ends at the navel.
5. The *yangyumei* begins at a point on the *dumei* at about the middle of the upper back and traverses the back of each arm and through the inside of the middle finger. The *Yangyumei* ends at the *laogong* point on the palm

of the hand. When you curl your fingers, the laogong point is where your middle finger rests against the palm.

6. The *yinyumei* meridian begins at the *laogong* points, traveling up the inside of each arm, across the pectoral muscles and through the nipples. The *Yinyumei* ends at the renmei after traveling a short distance along the daimei.

7. Beginning at the perineum and traveling along the front of each leg are the meridians called the *Yangqiaomei*. These meridians run the full length of the leg through the instep to the sole of the foot.

8. From the soles of the feet, the *yinqiaomei* move up the inside of each foot, looping around the ankles and returning to the perineum by way of the inner thighs.

The Junction Points

Impediments to the natural flow of energy are most likely to occur at the junction points. For that reason it is important to learn where these points are and to give them special attention while performing the exercises and using acupressure points.

At a point between the legs and halfway from the genitals to the anus is the junction of the yangyumei, the yinqiaomei, the renmei, the dumei, and the chongmei. This is called the *huiyin*. *Mingmen* is at a point on the dumei directly behind the navel. At a point along the dumei between the shoulder and behind the heart is the *gaohuang*. This junction point is considered crucial for the health of the heart and lungs. In the middle of the top of the head is a point called the *niyuan*, which connects the chongmei with the dumei. The laogong, you may recall from the meridian list, is that spot on your palm where the middle finger rests when you curl your fingers. This is the point at which the *yangyumei* and the *yinyumei* meet. The *yangyumei* and the *yinyumei* meet at the laogong point. The navel itself is called *shenque* and is the junction point for the renmei and the daimei. The seventh junction point is called the *yongquan* and is on the sole of each foot about two-thirds of the way between the heel and the middle toe. This is the point at which the yangqiaomei meets the yinqiaomei.

Don't allow the Chinese names of these junction points and meridians to confuse you. It isn't necessary to memorize the names and learn how to pronounce them. The important thing to remember is approximately where the meridians and the junction points are located so that you can concentrate your thoughts on a particular area or pathway. For example, the exercise Bird's Feathered Hand involves the use of the arms and hands only. You will need only, then, to concentrate on the meridian that runs down the outside of your arm through the middle finger, the junction point, laogong, and the meridian that returns the energy back to the shoulder and trunk on the inside of your arm. The exercise called An, however, requires a twist of the waist. In that case, you will need to add the meridian that circles your waist to your list of targeted pathways. A diagram of all the meridians and junction points can be found in Appendix A. Use this diagram to help you identify and target the appropriate areas of your body as you practice your exercises.

The Benefits of Seated T'ai Chi

Seated T'ai Chi has proven to be a beneficial form of exercise. Students have come to me with reports of improvements in the range of their arm and shoulder movements, more flexibility in the their legs, an increase in lung capacity and fewer falls. At the end of each and every class, all of us are relaxed and refreshed.

One of the most impressive stories from my experience teaching T'ai Chi involves Kathleen, an eighty-nine-year-old woman who has lived in an assisted-living community for five years. During that time she has been an active participant in the exercise classes, both the dance and martial arts–based program and the seated T'ai Chi program.

She recounts how active she and her husband were in retirement up until the point at which he became ill. They golfed several times a week and took 4-mile walks each morning before breakfast. She was also an avid gardener, but during the last year of her husband's life, all of her time was occupied with his care.

After her husband's death, she spent months straightening out their business and financial affairs. As a result, her own physical condition deteriorated drastically. By the time she moved into the community, she was unable to do many simple tasks for herself such as putting on a coat, reaching for a light switch that was just above shoulder level, or putting curlers in the back of her hair. Though she used no aids such as a walker or a cane, she describes her legs as being "as hard and unyielding to the touch as PVC pipe." Her toes had become completely frozen so that she could not curl them and she was unable to walk the halls of the facility without stopping frequently to rest her legs. She often found herself short of breath walking from her apartment to the dining room or to an activity.

After three years of a forty-five-minute dance/martial arts standing exercise class, she noticed an improvement in the flexibility of her arms and shoulders. She was able to reach behind herself to slip her arms into the sleeves of a coat, the light switch in her apartment was no longer out of reach, and she could put curlers in the back of her hair. Oddly enough, however, there appeared to be no marked improvement in the strength or flexibility of her legs and she continued to be both breathless and in pain when walking more than a short distance.

Since completing one year in the *seated* T'ai Chi class, this woman is now able to curl her toes, raise her foot onto the ball, pull back her toes and circle her ankles. Additionally, her knee joints are flexible and her feeling of breathlessness is gone. On a recent visit with her son, she informed me that she was able to walk in the mall from store to store without stopping and without pain. Kathleen's story is an example of how powerful seated exercise can be. Her legs became stronger from T'ai Chi in a chair than they did from the standing dance and martial-arts exercise programs!

Proof That T'ai Chi Is Good for You

In answer to the increasing interest in alternative medicine and a burgeoning enrollment in T'ai Chi classes, a number of studies have been conducted to determine whether or not these methods, though long accepted by the Chinese, have any validity by our Western standards. The results of these studies are strikingly similar to my own experiences with my students. All of the studies show marked improvement in the sense of balance, blood-pressure levels, flexibility and muscle strength, peak oxygen intake, and body-fat percentages. Though all of the studies to date have involved the use of standing T'ai Chi exercises, it is my belief based on observing my students' results that a program such as the one described in this book would prove to be as beneficial in the long run as those that are the subject of current research.

Western research is limited in scope by the very nature of the science itself. In order to produce the requisite amount of quantitative data, all studies are restricted by several factors: number and type of subject divided into two groups, an experimental group and a control group, the interest of the researcher, and the interests of the funding source that underwrites the cost of the research. Studies that have been conducted into the effectiveness of T'ai Chi have limited their concentration to one or two measurable areas such as blood pressure or blood pressure and aerobic capacity.

The Taoist way of gaining scientific knowledge, on the other hand, is through observation and intuition. Methods of treatment such as acupuncture and acupressure resulted from listening to the stories of soldiers who had been cured of chronic pain and illness. After being pelted with rocks or pierced by arrows, many of these warriors experienced relief from the symptoms of injury and disease. Further experimentation led to the discovery of meridians and their juncture points with specific descriptions of their locations and connections to internal organs, joints, or muscle groups. Though not measurable because they are not visible, the existence of these pathways was established by the resultant cures on a variety of patients. Blows from rocks were substituted in practice with the less drastic but equally effective use of finger pressure while piercing was accomplished with the use of needles.

T'ai Chi Lowers Blood Pressure

Possibly because high blood pressure is a common disease among those over fifty, several of the clinical studies judged the merits of T'ai Chi exercise based on the beginning and ending blood-pressure levels of the subjects. For example, there was a study conducted at Johns Hopkins University in which half of the subjects were involved in a moderately intense aerobic exercise program. The other half participated in a T'ai Chi class. In this study, only aerobic capacity and blood-pressure levels were measured, and many of those who participated had elevated blood-pressure levels at the beginning of the program. The results of the study reveals that only those who used aerobics for their exercise program showed a marked improvement in their aerobic capacity, which was to be expected. However, both the aerobic group and the T'ai Chi group showed lower blood pressure at the end of the study. Although the aerobic capacity improved significantly only within the aerobic group, the reduction in blood-pressure levels was as substantial in the T'ai Chi group as in the aerobic group. My eighty-nine-year-old student whose flexibility has improved so much through the practice of T'ai Chi also has a history of high blood pressure. This condition has been controlled over the years with prescription medications. Although her blood pressure has been kept within the acceptable range, her levels were still higher than normal. That is no longer the case. Her last several blood-pressure readings have fallen comfortably within the normal range.

T'ai Chi Makes You Strong

In addition to the improvement in blood-pressure levels exhibited by the subjects of these clinical trials, a report by Paul Cerrato in the *RN* journal shows a threefold improvement in the health of older adults who were given an exercise routine of ten sets of T'ai Chi movements over a fifteen-week period. These subjects showed not only a marked reduction in blood-pressure levels but also a decrease in the incidence of falls and an increase in muscle strength for those with osteoarthritis.

Irene is another of my students in the assisted-living community. She is a woman in her mid-eighties who used to be subject to frequent falls. Her doctor suggested that she use a wheelchair to get around and she believed that she would be confined to that chair for the rest of her life. However, since participating regularly in our seated T'ai Chi classes, her legs have strengthened sufficiently to allow her to walk around. Irene also has diabetes but is no longer dependent on either insulin shots or pills. She is healthier and happier now and a confirmed T'ai Chi enthusiast.

In another study described by Cathy Kessenich in *Orthopaedic Nursing*, nine experienced T'ai Chi practitioners were compared in the performance of five balance tests against nine nonpractitioners. The T'ai Chi group far surpassed the others in postural control. Additionally, this report cites a large study completed in 1996, in which subjects in a treatment group practiced T'ai Chi regularly three to four times a week over a twelve-year period. Compared to sedentary people in the same age group, the T'ai Chi practitioners showed a greater peak oxygen uptake and greater flexibility, which would reduce the number of falls since stiffness and pain in the knee, hip, and ankle joints is often the reason for falls among elderly people. Of importance for all age groups, this same study indicated that T'ai Chi caused a reduction in the percentage of body fat.

The research is continuing, particularly with subjects over the age of sixty. What has piqued the interest of these medical researchers, though the results are still preliminary, is the remarkable improvement in the general condition and well-being of the subjects. In several cases, medical investigators are recommending T'ai Chi as a complement to more orthodox therapies.

Getting Started

Because T'ai Chi is truly a holistic approach to exercise, the surroundings, music, clothing, and time of day are considered by the Chinese to be of equal importance. T'ai Chi is generally practiced in the early morning and around sunset in the evening. If at all possible, this is a good way to plan your practice times.

T'ai Chi is customarily performed outdoors in a park. Your own yard would be an ideal place, weather permitting. If none of those are possible because of the difficulty in getting outside, setting yourself up outdoors with a chair, or if you live in an urban area with a great deal of traffic and noise, consider what is available to you within your own home or apartment. Pick a favorite room, preferably one with a good sized window that looks out on a pleasant scene.

To further enhance the mood of your surroundings, you may want to use music to accompany the exercises. Some good choices, all specifically composed for use with T'ai Chi, are listed in Appendix B. If you have a piece of music that you like, use it. But choose carefully. Anything that is too fast, has lyrics, or is too heavy on the rhythm will distract you from concentrating on your movements and breath and may lead you to speed up exercises that are meant to be performed slowly and thoughtfully.

Another addition to the room that you might consider is a tabletop fountain or waterfall. These are available in many department stores, art galleries, or through catalogues. The sound of water is soothing and will aid in the calming of the spirit that we are seeking through our practice of T'ai Chi.

Remember always to wear loose, comfortable clothing, nothing that binds or constricts you in your movements. Since these exercises are of the seated variety, the question of footwear is of little importance as long as your shoes don't pinch your feet.

While these are considered the ideal conditions in which to practice T'ai Chi, the pace of our lives doesn't always permit us the luxury of peaceful, meditative sessions twice a day. Chapter 4, therefore, describes fifteen-minute exercise routines that will be as effective as the complete routine if practiced consistently and with concentration. These exercises can be performed at your desk at the office or at home. You probably already have plants somewhere in your office. Tabletop fountains or waterfalls are available in a variety of sizes so no matter how small the space, you may be able to find one that will be just the right size. Bring a portable CD or tape player to use while you exercise. If there is a window close to your desk that has a pleasant view, face it as you begin your session.

Each of these short sessions begins with deep diaphragmatic breathing to oxygenate your whole system. You will find that the breathing exercises alone will make a considerable difference to how you feel the rest of the day since indoor air quality in office buildings and in many homes is usually poor. The exercises for day one target the internal organs while days two and three are designed to strengthen and flex the muscles and joints of the upper body. The lower-body exercises from the complete routine are divided equally between day four and day five. Each of the sessions ends with a portion of the complete relaxation exercises and acupressure points that address a number of common complaints. Chapter 4 lists many additional acupressure points and you may wish to substitute or add those that may be more helpful for you.

Posture and the alignment of the body are so important in properly performing exercises of any kind that I have included a reminder at the beginning of each section. Imagine for a moment—or try it out if you can—that you are lying on your back. If your legs are stretched out, there will be a curvature in your back at about the midpoint. If you bend your knees, you are unable to slip your hand between the floor and your back because when you bent your knees, your spine became perfectly flat. This is the posture that you want while you are exercising. For our purposes, this means that you will have to pay particular attention to tucking your hips under a bit in order to press the small of your back against the back of your chair. It is best to have a chair with a solid back and one high enough to support your entire back while you are exercising. Before you begin the following exercises on the next page or those comprising day one of the fifteen-minute exercise routines, close your eyes for a moment, take several deep breaths and sink gently into the contours of your chair.

The Complete Routine

After a time of decay comes the turning point.
The powerful light that has been banished returns.
There is movement, but it is not brought about by force.
The movement is natural, arising spontaneously.
For this reason the transformation of the old becomes easy.
The old is discarded and the new is introduced.
Both measures accord with the time; therefore no harm results.

—I CHING

"At my last birthday party, I surprised everyone by blowing out all the candles on the cake. My daughter wanted to know how I was able to do it. And, I told her it's because of the breathing exercises we do in the T'ai Chi class. I said maybe she ought to try it." Peggy was celebrating her ninety-third birthday on that occasion and continues to attend class four times a week. She isn't the only student who has had some remarkable things to say about the improvement in their physical and mental well-being. Of course, not all of them are over ninety years of age! Nevertheless, their enthusiasm for the results of this program equal, and sometimes surpass, Peggy's own experience.

How T'ai Chi Works

There is really nothing too surprising about successful results from the practice of T'ai Chi for T'ai Chi is truly a simple, nonstressful, and most importantly, *holistic* exercise system. All of the movements are based on the theory that the human body contains a system of pathways along which energy travels as it nourishes and heals muscles, bones, and organs. Because Chinese philosophy teaches that body, mind, and spirit are really one, the movement of ch'I, or energy, traversing the body brings not only physical healing but also mental and spiritual benefits as well. In the Oriental view, we are not a collection of body parts, a mind, and a soul that just happen to be bound together in one space but rather a seamless web of all that defines each of us as an individual. Nor are we are individuals standing all alone, like islands separated from each other by miles of water. Rather, we are symbiotic or mutually and beneficially dependent entities within that greater seamless web that is the cosmos.

That web of internal and external forces may help to explain why you do not feel particularly well or vital. Environmental factors such as indoor air pollution or any number of the toxic chemicals found outdoors, stresses at home and at work, poor dietary habits, a sedentary lifestyle, and so on all contribute to our feelings of physical, mental, and spiritual unease.

In the process of performing these T'ai Chi exercises, you will be mentally activating that energy that exists naturally in your body. As you stimulate the ch'i along the meridians, breaking up the obstructions caused by the previously mentioned factors, toxins will be pushed along those pathways and circulated throughout the body. Our next job, then, is to remove these toxins entirely from the body The only way to effectively remove them is by drinking water—lots and lots of water.

The Importance of Water

At a conservative estimate, water comprises 75 percent of the human body. Brain tissue is believed to be 85 percent water. Current studies indicate that an adult, in order to be properly hydrated, requires at least half a gallon of water (fruit juice may be substituted for a portion of the water) per day. If you weigh over 200 pounds, an additional 8-ounce glass of water for every

10 pounds over 200 pounds is necessary to prevent dehydration. Dehydration is seldom recognized for what it is. Most of us assume we don't need to drink any water unless we experience dryness in the mouth. The need for water to replenish the body's tissues occurs well before our mouths feel dry. Additionally, many of us have the habit of drinking coffee and/or caffeinated soft drinks all day long. The overuse of these products may be dulling our ability to measure when we are dehydrated. The caffeine in coffee and in most soft drinks not only destroys the water contained within them but also depletes the body's reserves of water.

Hydration, however, is not our only concern here. Because we are using T'ai Chi exercises to rid our bodies of toxins, we must also consider the importance of flushing them thoroughly so that these same toxins will not remain trapped in the meridians or in the juncture points where the meridians come together. Keep a glass or a waterbottle handy. As you go through the exercises, take a good healthy sip of water at the end of each section or whenever your mouth feels dry. Don't worry about extra trips to the bathroom. Frequent urination may mean you are ridding your body of toxins more quickly than you ordinarily do. Bear in mind, also, that if you have not been drinking this much water, your body will need some time to adjust to the increase in fluids. Once that occurs, the frequency of urination will naturally be reduced.

Before You Start

On the succeeding pages of this chapter there is a thorough description of the seated T'ai Chi exercises. It will take approximately fifty to sixty minutes to finish the entire set, including the introductory breathing exercises. You may reduce the number of repetitions in order to complete the exercises in less time or you may wish to consult Chapter 5 for daily exercises that will take you approximately fifteen minutes to complete. Whichever set of exercises you decide to do, be consistent. If your schedule doesn't allow for an hour of uninterrupted time to complete the full exercise program, then use the fifteen-minute sets instead. Most importantly, don't start out with a bang and end with a whimper. There is nothing that defeats any exercise system more often than a rush of enthusiasm at the beginning that is too overwhelming and time-consuming to be maintained over a period of months and years. T'ai Chi was designed to be practiced as any other daily habit such as brushing your teeth or combing your hair. If at all possible, try to do your exercises twice a day, once in the morning and once in the evening before you go to bed. You will perform your duties throughout the day with more vigor and enthusiasm. You will accomplish more in one day than you ever imagined possible, and at night, you'll sleep like a baby!

Breathing Exercises

Breath is essential for life, yet we breathe without conscious thought. Unless we make an effort to practice deep breathing, we are all breathing in a shallow way. According to Dennis Lewis, the founder of Authentic Breathing Resources, proper respiration (that is, deep, diaphragmatic breathing) may be the single most effective tool against asthma, poor digestion, weight gain, sleeplessness, high blood pressure, heart disease, stress, and a multitude of other ailments brought about by our modern lifestyle. Deep, conscious breathing cleanses the body and boosts the immune system. How we breathe affects our metabolism because it is *oxygen* that activates the metabolic process that breaks down the fats into carbon dioxide and water, which are then expelled as waste. Of the forty-two pints of fluids that circulate throughout the body every day nourishing and oxidizing the cells, six pints pass through the lymphatic system cleansing the body of excess proteins, waste products, and fats that would otherwise clog the tissues. The fats that remain in the body are utilized either for energy or are stored for future use. Too much stored fat depletes our energy resources and results in weight gain. For you and me this means that ignoring the way we breathe jeopardizes our health and practically guarantees that, unless our dietary habits are exemplary, we will gain and retain excess weight.

Healthy breathing also has a profound effect on our emotional state (consider the shortness of breath and tightness in the chest in moments of stress or fear). Deep breathing cleanses not only the body and its many organs and systems but also calms the emotions and heightens our spiritual and intuitive state. Memory and mental clarity can also be vastly improved if we can only teach ourselves to breathe in the right way.

In this section of exercises, we are going to concentrate not just on breathing but on *how* we breathe. For the purpose of clarity, we will define and visualize ch'i as a disc or ball and energy as the "sparks" thrown off by the momentum of the spinning disc. The basis of T'ai Chi is *nonaction* and for that reason, it is helpful to think of yourself purely as a bundle of bones without flesh or muscle. Though it may seem contradictory, while we are taking action and achieving our desired results, we are doing so in a *nonactive* way without straining muscles and stressing the body.

The first exercise in this section lays the groundwork for what follows by concentrating on the diaphragm as the breath enters through the nose and is exhaled through the mouth. Holding your hands lightly over the diaphragmatic area is a reminder of what is happening when you are breathing properly. Butterfly circulates the energy while Flower Bud Opens centers the chi and brings the entire body back into balance. Dragon's Breath warms the body giving you an extra burst of energy. Backward Arm Swings open the chest cavity allowing the air to move freely in and out of the lungs. This is a particularly good exercise for eliminating shortness of breath. Finally, Centering Chi returns the chi to its position in the lower dan tien, preventing it from becoming trapped in another part of the body.

In addition, before we start, we must center body, mind, and spirit in order to perform the following exercises for our maximum benefit. If you are doing your breathing exercises first thing in the morning, you'll want to clear your mind of any fuzziness or memories of unpleasant dreams. If you are doing these exercises in the evening, you'll want to rid yourself of the irritations and stresses experienced throughout the day. Begin to bring your whole self into balance by visualizing a rapidly flowing body of water. Imagine the ripples and waves as your day or night with its ups and downs. Concentrate on this image as you calm the waves until the water is as clear and smooth as glass. When you feel sufficiently relaxed and centered, begin the first exercise.

❧ Balloon Breathing

Benefits: Cleansing the lungs and strengthening the muscles of the diaphragm.

Posture: Begin by sitting with your back against the back of the chair. Legs should be shoulder-width apart, feet flat on the floor. Tuck your hips under slightly and curve your shoulders inward without hunching. the idea here is to keep the ch'i from flowing outward away from the body. Hold your head lightly on your neck as though it were suspended by a string from the ceiling.

Visualization: Imagine a disk that is ch'i. It is stationary and still. As you breathe in, set the disc in motion with your mind. As it begins to spin faster and faster, exhale and allow the sparks of energy to shoot through your body. Direct that energy upward through and around your trunk.

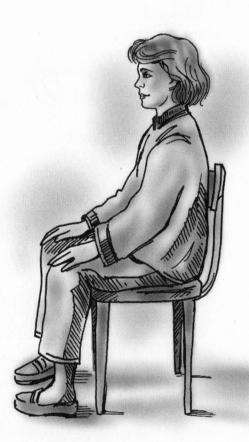

Posture

1. Close your eyes. Hold both hands over your diaphragm so that you can feel the muscles expanding and contracting as your breathe in and out.

2. Inhale deeply through your nose, expanding your diaphragm. The disc (ch'i) is located in the lower abdomen (lower dan tien) about three finger widths below your navel. By breathing in deeply, you have set that disc in motion. It begins to pick up speed and as it does, energy is released. It is your mind that determines where the energy will be sent so imagine the energy sparks traveling upward through your abdomen, into your chest where the sparks will circle in and out and around the lungs.

3. Exhale through your mouth and as you do so, envision the toxins that have collected in your lungs exiting through your mouth and out of your system.

Repetitions: Nine

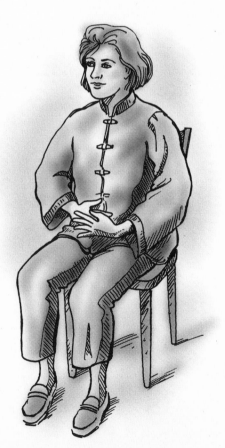

Balloon Breathing

∾ **Butterfly**

Benefits: Opening the chest to expand the lungs to their fullest extent.

Posture: As in the previous exercise.

Visualization: Imagine that you are swimming through molecules of air. You are both receiving and giving energy to your immediate surroundings. The area around you is not a void but, rather, is filled with densely packed molecules of air and electromagnetic energy.

Pathways: In this exercise, you are not only opening your chest to its limit but you are also drawing energy from the lower dan tien to the middle dan tien located at the level of your solar plexus. You are clearing away any obstructions that may be present, along the middle meridian that runs from the perineum through the middle of your body to the top of your head. Once the pathway is free of obstacles, the energy you have brought up from the lower *dan tien* will flow freely.

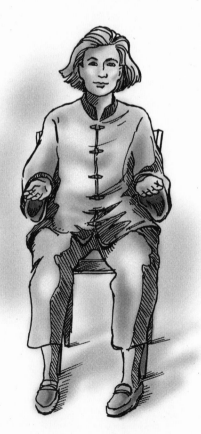

Butterfly

1. Begin with your hands at your waist. Move them forward and slightly upward until they are directly in front of your solar plexus.
2. Turn your palms back to back and push forward until your elbows are straight. As you move your arms forward, inhale deeply through your nose, expanding your diaphragm. Continue breathing in until your arms are as far in front of you as possible.
3. As you move your arms out to the side and behind you, exhale, tightening your diaphragm and abdominal muscles. Make sure that you are using your diaphragm, not your shoulders to move the air in and out of your lungs.

Repetitions: Nine

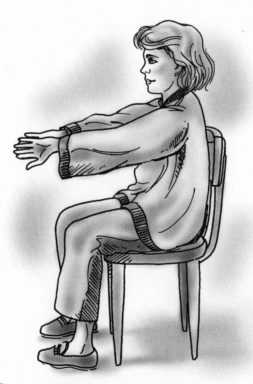

Butterfly (continued)

∽ **Flower Bud Opens**

Benefits: The chest opens to the fullest extent allowing for a deeper inhalation while lifting the rib cage.

Posture: Begin in the same position that you were in for the previous exercises. At the point where your arms move upward and over your head, arch your back away from the back of your chair until you begin to bring your arms out to the side and back to the front of your chest. Slowly press your back against your chair and tuck your hips underneath you.

Visualization: Think about the first yawn of the morning. It is deep, relaxing, and satisfying. Your chest opens wide as clean, clear air enters your lungs.

Pathways: In this exercise you are expanding your chest and lungs still further. Imagine that the energy that has been brought up through the center of your body is now extended to the upper dan tien at the top of your head. Energy is circulating through the shoulders, neck, head, and arms

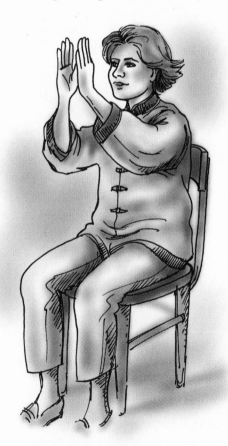

Flower Bud Opens

as well as through the meridian that runs up your spine. Obstructions along the front and back pathways are being cleared each time you stretch and inhale. You want to press the sparks of energy into the very marrow of your bones to cleanse and strengthen.

1. Raise your hands over your head with palms facing through the middle of your chest. There is tension here in your arms as you move them upward.
2. Press your arms down to the sides, palms facing the floor as you arch your back.
3. Bring your arms, completely relaxed again and loose, behind you and then return them to the front of your chest.
   Repetitions: Nine

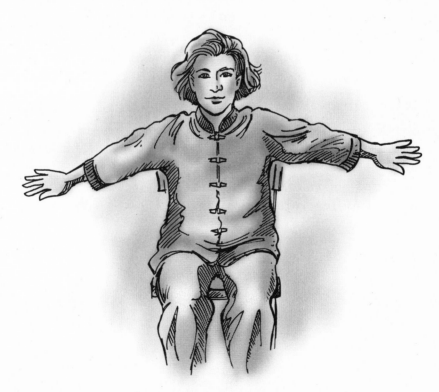

Flower Bud Opens (continued)

∾ Backward Arm Swings

Benefits: Strengthening and tightening of the arm muscles as well as opening the chest for deeper breathing.

Posture: As in the previous exercise.

Visualization: Imagine that you are pushing backward against a wall. That wall is made up of the molecules of air, and you are once again exchanging energy with your immediate surroundings.

Pathways: In this exercise you are opening your chest once again to increase the inward flow of fresh air and the expulsion of toxins that may be trapped in the alveoli, the small sacs at the bottom of your lungs. Any toxic substances that you have inhaled will remain in the alveoli unless your breathing is sufficiently deep to root them out and expel them as you exhale. In addition, the backward swinging of your arms propels the energy down the meridian on the outside of your arms, through the middle finger and the juncture point on your palm. The energy then moves back up to your shoulders through the pathway that runs up the inside of your arms. You should feel a definite tingling in your hands when you have completed this exercise.

1. Swing your arms backward with your palms facing the imaginary wall behind you.

2. You are expending energy as you push your arms backward but making no effort as your arms move forward with the momentum created by the backward motion.

   Repetitions: Twenty-seven, or three sets of nine.

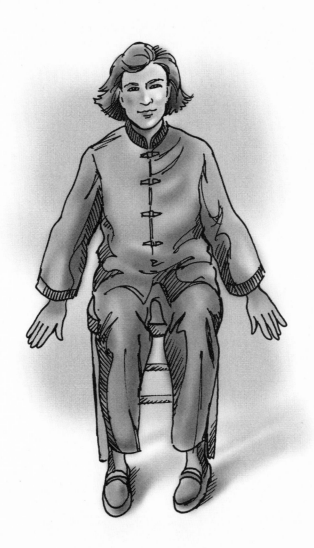

Backward Arm Swings

Benefits: Centers the energy and rebalances the body.

Posture: As in the previous exercise.

Visualization: Imagine that you are collecting the ch'i and bits of energy from all over your body returning them to a neutral position at the lower dan tien so that no energy will be lost or trapped elsewhere in the body.

Pathways: You are targeting all the pathways you have used in the previous exercises.

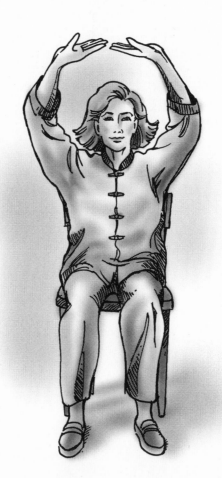

Centering Ch'i

1. Hold your hands, palm up, just above your lap. Breathe in deeply through your nose while contracting your diaphragm. In this exercise, the diaphragm is **not** expanded during inhalations.

2. As you tighten your diaphragm and abdomen, raise your arms out to the side and up over your head to its center. Your palms are now facing the ceiling, fingers barely touching.

3. Allow your arms to descend gradually in an arc out to the side. As you do so, exhale until there is no breath left in your lungs and relax the muscles of your diaphragm and abdomen.

4. Return your arms to the original position in front of the lowest part of your abdomen, palms facing upward.

   Repetitions: Three

   Relax for a moment before beginning the next set of exercises.

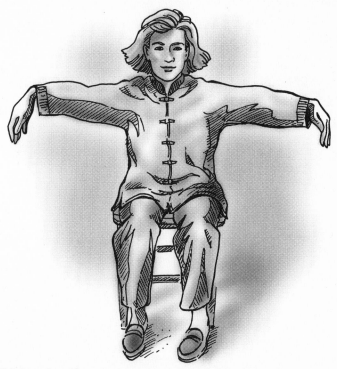

Centering Ch'i (continued)

～ Dragon's Breath

Benefits: For quick energy, stimulation of circulation, cleansing of the nasal passages, and tightening of the abdominal muscles.

Posture: Begin by sitting with your back against the back of the chair. Legs should be shoulder-width apart, feet flat on the floor. Tuck your hips under slightly and curve your shoulders inward without hunching. Hold your head lightly on your neck as though it were suspended by a string from the ceiling.

Visualization: Imagine that you are stoking a boiler. As you breathe rapidly in and out you are fanning the fire of your circulatory system.

Pathways: This movement sends energy through all the meridians of the trunk and arms quickly because of the force of the inhalations and exhalations.

1. Breathe in slowly through your nose, expanding your diaphragm. Exhale slowly through your mouth.
   Repetitions: Three

2. Inhale and exhale rapidly as though you were sneezing or blowing your nose. Repeat the quick breaths.
   Repetitions: Eighteen

3. Gradually slow your breathing down with a slight pause between the inhale and the exhale.
   Repetitions: Six

Healing Exercises

The early Taoists viewed the human body as a microcosm of the universe. As mentioned, the Taoists believed that the body contains circuits of energy that flow incessantly not through nerves or blood vessels but through invisible pathways called meridians. These pathways meet at certain junction points which, along with the entire span of the meridians, may become blocked. The pathways and junctures comprise a self-contained, closed system, either intersecting with each other or beginning or ending with other meridians. As a result, blockage of one pathway may also affect at least one other pathway or junction point. We may not know exactly where each and every blockage has occurred, but by following the order of the exercises, every meridian and junction will receive our attention at some point and we will be able to release whatever impediments exist.

Similar to the way we regard our breathing, we tend to ignore our internal organs as long as they appear to be functioning normally. Like any other components of the body, however, they too require stimulation and attention if they are to operate at their maximum efficiency. By the time a problem has arisen, it may be too late to begin paying attention to these vital organs.

We are going to begin again with a check of our posture. Make certain that you are seated with your legs shoulder-width apart, feet pointing in a bit, and shoulders hunched ever so slightly. As you perform the exercises, relax your torso so that you are able to turn fully from the waist. Concentrate on the area of the body that is being squeezed and massaged along with the meridians and junctions that are located in that region. We will be repeating an equal number of movements on each side so that if you wish to reduce the number of repetitions or increase them, you must make certain that you keep the number of movements consistent on the left and the right sides.

If you have lost your feeling of calm and concentration between the two exercise sections, repeat one of the breathing exercises or once again visualize the cessation of the ripples and waves of your imaginary river. Whichever you choose to do, remember the effort put forth in T'ai Chi is more mental than physical. There should be no excessive strain on the muscles in any of these movements but rather an application of thought and a steady concentration of the will on the targeted area.

∾ **White Crane**

Benefits: Energizing all the organs in the trunk and reducing the waistline.

Posture: Begin by sitting with your back against the back of the chair. Legs should be shoulder-width apart, feet flat on the floor. Tuck your hips under slightly and curve your shoulders inward without hunching. Hold your head lightly on your neck as though it were suspended by a string from the ceiling.

Visualization: Imagine that you are squeezing and massaging your internal organs, exercising them by twisting your trunk and breathing deeply.

Pathways: In this exercise, the pathway receiving the most stimulation is the one that circles your waist.

1. Begin with your right hand alongside your right ear, palm forward. Press your left arm downward, palm held horizontal with the floor.

2. Twist from the waist to your left bringing your right arm around to your left side until your right hand is parallel and about 4 or 5 inches from your left ear.

3. As you turn back to center, sweep your right arm across your trunk and raise your left hand palm forward alongside your left ear. Swing to your right, pressing your right hand downward so that your right palm is facing the floor while remaining and horizontal.

4. As you twist from the waist, your left hand will move with you. Finish with the left hand about 4 or 5 inches from your right ear, palm facing your back.

5. Breathe in through your nose when you are facing forward and out through your mouth as you turn to each side. These will not be deep breaths because the twisting motion will prevent you from expanding your diaphragm as far as you did in the previous exercises.

   Repetitions: Eighteen times, or nine times in each direction.

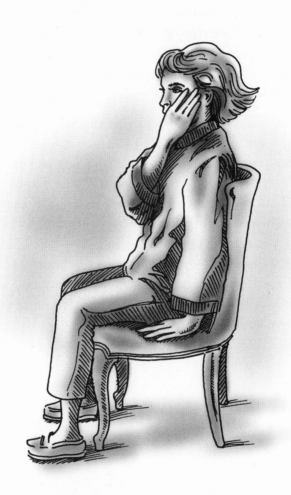

White Crane

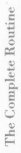

↶ Push Up Sky/Press Down on Earth

Benefits: Stretches the arm muscles and slims the waistline.

Posture: As in the previous exercise.

Visualization: Imagine that you are creating a space between the sky and the earth and, by touching each, you are connecting with the energies of both.

Pathways: Think of the energy flowing into your trunk from the lower dan tien, through your shoulders, and up and down your arms traveling through all the pathways of your trunk, neck, and head, as well as those in the shoulders and arms.

1. Begin with your hands resting on your thighs.
2. Bring your right arm up with the palm facing the ceiling and at the same time press downward with your left hand, palm facing to the floor. Breathe in through your nose and expand your diaphragm.
3. Bring both arms, elbows bent, to the level of your solar plexus. Breathe out through your mouth. Tighten your diaphragm and abdomen and hold until you need to breathe in again.
4. Reverse your hands so that the left one reaches toward the ceiling this time and the right is pressing downward. Continue alternating sides, breathing in deeply as one arm ascends and the other descends.

Repetitions: Eighteen, or two sets of nine.

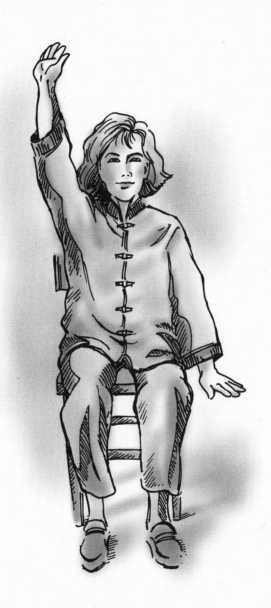

Push Up Sky/Press Down on Earth

∾ Turtle

Benefits: Stretches neck and shoulder muscles and strengthens the muscles of the abdomen and the diaphragm.

Posture: As in the previous exercises.

Visualization: Imagine that you are a turtle poking your head and legs out of your shell.

Pathways: As you breathe in and stretch, think of the energy flowing from your trunk into your neck and head and downward into your arms.

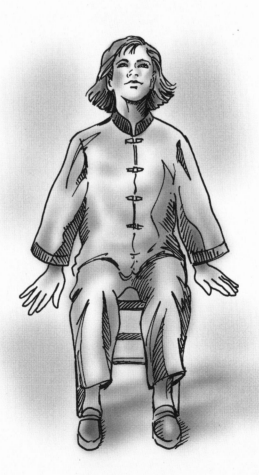

Turtle

1. Begin again with your hands resting on your thighs.

2. Stretch your neck and press down on your shoulders while turning your palms toward the floor and keeping them horizontal to the floor. Bend your head back slightly and look up at the ceiling. Breathe in through your nose while expanding your diaphragm.

3. As your breathe out through your mouth, bend your head downward a bit and bring your arms in front of your abdomen as though you were retreating into your shell. Contract your abdomen as strongly as you are able.

Repetitions: Nine

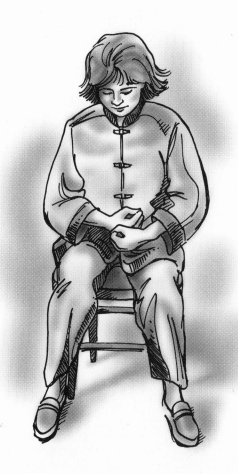

Turtle (continued)

Benefits: Circulates the energy, stretching the arm and shoulder muscles.

Posture: As in the previous exercises.

Visualization: Your hands are touching the heavens and your feet are planted firmly on the earth. You are a conduit of their energies, exchanging and receiving ch'i.

Pathways: Think about the energy circulating throughout your internal organs, moving up and down your arms, through your neck and head.

1. Lace your fingers and swing your arms over your head to its center, palms facing the ceiling. Remember to breathe in deeply using your diaphragm. Do not lift your shoulders when you bring your arms over your head. Press down on your shoulders and stretch just the muscles of your arms.

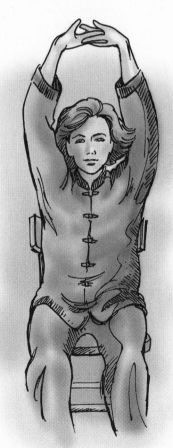

Holding Up Sky

2. Bring your arms back down as your breathe out and tighten your abdomen.
Repetitions: Nine
3. On the ninth upward movement, lean to your right, then your left, and so on from the waist only. On the last count, you will be leaning to your right.
Repetitions: Nine
4. Swing your arms out in front of your chest or clockwise back to the center of your head and continue circling. Then repeat the leans beginning on the left.
Repetitions: Nine

(continued)

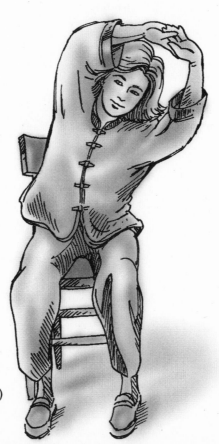

Holding Up Sky (continued)

5. On the ninth lean, circle again moving in the opposite direction or counterclockwise.
   Repetitions: Nine
6. Repeat the up and down swings. Stop and rest your arms.
   Repetitions: Nine

Each time your swing your arms up over your head, breathe in through your nose and expand your diaphragm. When your arms return to your lap, breathe out and tighten your abdomen. Breathe lightly as you lean from side to side but deeply just before you begin to circle your arms and then expel the breath as you lean forward. There should be a slight pause at the top of the revolution to give you time to inhale completely.

∾ An

Benefits: Exercises the internal organs and stretches shoulder and arm muscles.

Posture: As in the previous exercises.

Visualization: Think of your hands pressing against the molecules of air as an exchange of energy with your immediate surroundings.

Pathways: Energy moves from the daimei at your waist, through the trunk, and into your arms. As you return your arms to your shoulders, you are bringing the energy along the meridian on the inside of your arm back to the trunk.

Think of this as you perform the exercise—the Chinese word *an* refers to the type of pressure used by an experienced massage therapist. Use just the right amount of force, but don't overdo it.

1. Hold your hands palm forward in front of your shoulders. Twist to your left and push your arms out to the side until your elbows are nearly straight.
2. Bring your arms back in front of your shoulders, breathe in, twist to your left, and push your arms out as you exhale.

Repetitions: Eighteen, or nine pushes to each side.

∞ Brushing Tree Trunk

Benefits: Loosens and flexes neck muscles while balancing the right and left hemispheres of the brain.

Posture: As in the previous exercises.

Visualization: Once again, imagine the twisting motions in this exercise squeezing and massaging the internal organs.

Pathways: Think about the energy as it circulates through the meridians of the trunk, in and around all the organs.

1. Extend your arms and reach for the ceiling. Take a deep breath expanding your diaphragm.

2. Swing your right arm down across your chest to your left side. The left arm remains stretched toward the ceiling.

3. As your right arm wraps around your waist on the left side, turn your head so you are looking to your right. In other words, your body is twisted to the left but your head is turned in the opposite direction. Breathe out as you bend forward and tighten your abdomen.

4. Swing your right arm up again and reverse the rotation so that your left arm is resting on your right hip. Turn your head to the left. Exhale as you bend over and twist. Breathe in at the center point.

Repetitions: Eighteen, or nine times twisting to each side.

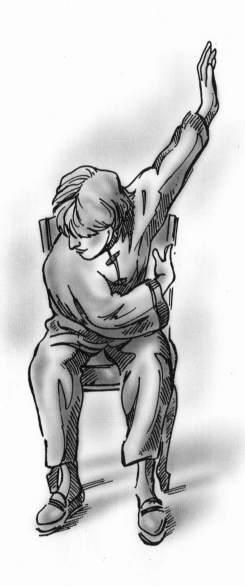

Brushing Tree Trunk

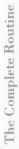

Benefits: Restores balance and renews energy.

Posture: As in the previous exercises.

Visualization: Picture all of the energy returning from various parts of your body. The energy is being pulled back into the disc at the lower dan tien from which it came. None has been lost or trapped and balance is restored.

Pathways: You are targeting all the pathways you have used in the previous exercises.

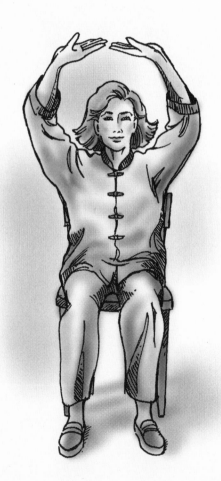

Centering Ch'i

1. Hold your hands palm up, just above your lap. Breathe in deeply through your nose while contracting your diaphragm. In this exercise, the diaphragm is **not** expanded during inhalations.

2. As you tighten your diaphragm and abdomen, raise your arms out to the side and up over your head to its center. Your palms are now facing the ceiling, fingers barely touching.

3. Allow your arms to descend gradually in an arc out to the side. As you do so, exhale until there is no breath left in your lungs and relax the muscles of your diaphragm and abdomen.

4. Return your arms to the original position in front of the lowest part of your abdomen, palms facing upward.

   Repetitions: Three

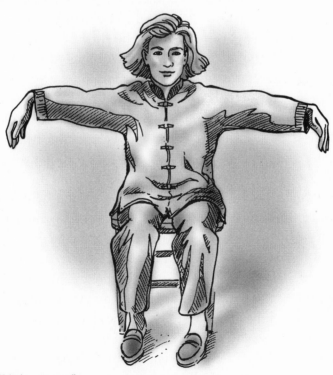

Centering Ch'i (continued)

Upper-Body Exercises

In the previous section we were concerned with squeezing and stimulating the internal organs. Now, we are going to concentrate on both loosening and strengthening the joints, bones, and muscles of the upper body. None of the following exercises is strenuous. Although muscles are tightened and then relaxed, at no time should there be excessive strain. As in all of these T'ai Chi movements, relaxation is the key. Remember that these are *mental* exercises—the mind is actively seeking to stimulate the flow of energy in and through the muscles and joints of the upper body. That is not accomplished by stressing your muscles or joints but rather by using your mind to move the sparks from the spinning disc (ch'i) through the meridians of the trunk. These meridians include the one that runs up the spine and over the head. The second pathway runs downward from the tip of the tongue back to the perineum. The meridian that circles your waist and the one that runs straight through the center of your body from the perineum to the top of your head are the other two pathways you will need to concentrate on during these exercises. Arm movements will stimulate the flow of energy through the meridian on the outside of your arm and back through the meridian on the inside of the arm that returns energy to the trunk.

Five of the juncture points are also located in the upper body. There is one junction point directly behind the navel called the *mingmen* and another between the shoulder blades and behind the heart called the *gaohuang*. The third junction point is in the middle of the very top of the head (the *niyuan*); while the fourth is located on the palm (the *laogong*). The fifth junction point is the navel (the *shenque*). These will be points of concentration at different times while you are performing the exercises.

The first set of exercises relaxes and loosens the head, neck, and shoulders. This involves the upper dan tien and the last section of the pathway known as the *dumei*, which runs upward along the spine. Concentrate on the beginning of the pathway that returns down the front of the body called the *renmei* and the uppermost part of the channel that rises from the perineum, directly through the center of the body to the top of the head as you perform the exercises. With the inclusion of shoulder shrugs and drops, visualize both the outer arm meridian at its point of origin and the inner arm meridian at its end. If you have any respiratory problems, whether chronic or temporary, you will want to concentrate particularly on the *gaohuang* junction point located directly behind the heart. A weak heart muscle or palpitations may be due to the absence of sufficient energy flow through this junction.

Wild Horse centers the body when the hands are placed in front of the chest and a deep breath is taken into the lungs. Leans to each side gently stretch the arm, back, and side muscles as you exhale. There is an additional exercise for your eyes in Wild Horse if you follow the movement of your hand as it is lifted up and out to the side.

Bird's Feathered Hand should draw your attention to the spatial relationship between your arm and the air surrounding it. You will increase the strength of your grip through the isometric exercise of closing your hand as though there were a hard ball or some other form of resistance between your fingers and your palm. Bursitis, stiff shoulders or fingers, pain in your arms or hands may indicate a blockage somewhere along the yangyumei or yinyumei or possibly at the laogong junction. It is all right to increase the repetitions in these areas if you feel they need more attention. However, don't overdo. Consistency in exercising will eventually resolve some of these problems, not an excessive work out all at one time. Remember that your arms and your hands are completely relaxed during this movement until you begin to close your hand around the imaginary obstruction.

Hands Waving in Clouds is a soft movement with no strain whatsoever. This exercise should relax any muscles that have become overly taut during Bird's Feathered Hand. You will be rotating at the waist, stretching those muscles, and trimming your waistline as a result.

The exercise known as Green Dragon moves the energy from shoulder and ear to the center of your body as you bring your arms across your chest ending with one hand in a knife position and the other brushing the top of your thigh. In this movement, too, your arms are completely relaxed until you reach the end of the downward motion. At that point, you stiffen both arms and exhale.

Repulse Monkey is a rather vicious attack when T'ai Chi is used as a martial art. For our purposes, *Repulse Monkey* is a wonderful example of the multiplicity of benefits contained in each of the T'ai Chi exercises. Shoulder muscles are loosened gently by the swing of your working arm. Looking over your shoulder as you swing your arm up and over stretches your neck muscles. Following the movement of the arm will exercise your eyes and enhance your peripheral vision.

Plucking Thread is another arm, shoulder, and eye exercise. Pulling up the arm while keeping your shoulder level tightens the muscles at the back of arms, reducing or preventing flabby upper arms. It is a very gentle way of toning your triceps.

In the Trunk Rotation exercise, your attention should again be focused on the placement and activity of the ch'i at the lower dan tien. Breathing in and expanding your diaphragm while upright encourages more ch'i activity resulting in another burst of energy through your system. As an added bonus, hip joints are loosened and abdominal muscles are tightened as you swing your trunk down and around.

◁ Head, Neck, and Shoulders

Benefits: Relaxes the muscles of the neck and realigns the cervical vertebrae.

Posture: Begin by sitting with your back against the back of the chair. Legs should be shoulder-width apart, feet flat on the floor. Tuck your hips under slightly and curve your shoulders inward without hunching. Hold your head lightly on your neck as though it were suspended by a string from the ceiling.

Visualization: Imagine that your neck muscles are as supple as an infant's and that your head is a light ball perched on a flexible stalk.

Pathways: Remember that the neck is considered to be the link between the body and the mind. Tension in this area may indicate a conflict between thought and action. For those of us who spend a great deal of time at a desk and at a computer, tense neck muscles may be nothing more than the result of a static position held for too long. This exercise will ease the tension in your neck and shoulders by sending energy to the meridians in the back, front, and center of your neck. At the same time, any stress that has settled in the head or shoulders will be released.

Warning: Do not do this exercise if you have had surgery on your neck or a serious injury without first consulting your physician.

1. Breathe in while your head is upright.

2. Lower your head gently to your chest while breathing out.

3. Return your head to the center, breathing in again and lower it gently backwards as you breathe out.
Repetitions: Nine times, counting the forward and backward motion as one.

4. Now, let your head drop down toward your shoulder beginning on the right side.
Repetitions: Each lean to the side should be given one count for a total of nine.

5. You will finish with your head tilted to the right. Circle your head down to your chest and then back to the left. Do not lean your head backwards while circling.
Repetitions: Nine

6. Lean your head over your shoulder again beginning on the left.
Repetitions: Nine individual leans.

7. Circle your head from shoulder to chest to shoulder.
Repetitions: Nine

8. Look over your right shoulder and turn your eyes in the same direction as though you were trying to look at someone standing behind you. Now, glance over your left shoulder and continue alternating.
Repetitions: Nine swiveling movements.

9. Look over your left shoulder and tilt your head so that you are looking up into the corner where the wall and ceiling meet. Repeat on the right.
Repetitions: Alternate for nine head-turning lifts.

10. Raise your shoulders toward your ears. Allow them to drop abruptly. This is a particularly good exercise for stiff shoulders as long as there is no accompanying pain. If the shoulder drop is painful, lower your shoulders gently instead of dropping them.
Repetitions: Nine

11. Then, circle your shoulders backward. Breathe into the shoulder joint to make the rolling motion easier.
Repetitions: Nine

12. Now, circle your shoulders forward. Throughout all of these shoulder movements, allow your arms to dangle loosely by your sides.
Repetitions: Nine

∿ Wild Horse

Benefits: Helps to center the ch'i and stretches muscles along the sides of the trunk and the arms.

Posture: As in the previous exercise.

Visualization: As you hold the imaginary ball in front of you, picture the energy caught between your hands.

Pathways: As you move your hands out to the sides, imagine energy coursing through your arms and back again into the area defined by your hands. As you hold the imaginary ball in front of you, your hands are compressing the ch'i between the middle and lower dan tiens.

1. Hold your hands, palms together with your right hand on top and your left hand on the bottom, palm facing up. Your hands should be as far apart as they would be if you were holding a basketball. Your right hand will be at the level of your solar plexus, and your left hand at the level of your lower abdomen.

2. Now, bring your left hand from below your right and raise it to the side and up to eye level. Meanwhile, the right hand moves down and to the side with the palm facing the floor. Bring your left hand up and over your head as you lean to the right.

3. Return to the center and reverse your hands so that your left is now on top and your right is underneath. Make sure that your hands are as far apart as if you were holding a basketball.

4. Raise your right arm to the side and up to eye level as the left arm presses down and to the side. Lean over to the left and return to the center reversing your hands again.

Repetitions: Nine leans to each side, or a total of eighteen leans.

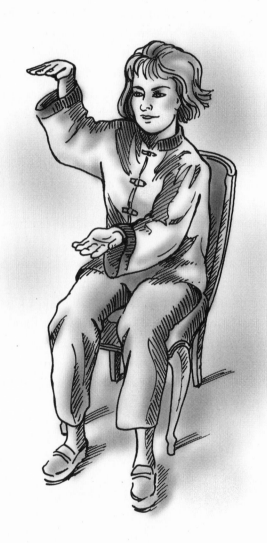

Wild Horse

Benefits: Strengthens the muscles of the forearm and hand, increasing the power of your grip.

Posture: As in the previous exercises.

Visualization: Imagine molecules of air passing between your fingers. As you close your hand, picture those molecules as solid matter that you must press flat making a tight fist.

Pathways: The energy will pass from your shoulders, down the outside of your arm through your middle finger to the juncture point on your palm. The force then returns to the shoulder by way of the meridian on the inside of your arm.

1. Fist your hands loosely in front of your shoulders.

2. Extend your right arm out to the side and as you do so, keep the arm and fingers relaxed.

3. Now, open your fingers as a bird's individual feathers spread when in flight.

4. Close your hand in a fist again, this time as tightly as you can. Hold for a moment and then relax your grip and the muscles of your arm as you return to the original position in front of your shoulder.

5. Repeat with the left hand. Don't forget that your hand and arm muscles should be relaxed at all times until the arm is completely extended. At that point, close your fist as tightly as you can and tense your arm muscles. Relax all the muscles again with your hand in a loose fist as you return your hand to the shoulder.

Repetitions: Nine extensions to each side for a total of eighteen.

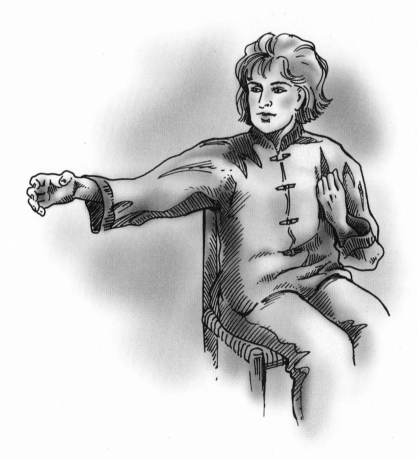

Bird's Feathered Hand

∽ Hands Waving in Clouds

Benefits: Strengthens shoulder and upper arm muscles and trims the waist.

Posture: As in the previous exercises.

Visualization: Imagine that you are brushing wisps of clouds from in front of your face, chest, and abdomen.

Pathways: The source of the energy in this exercise is the meridian at the waist called the daimei. Energy is released as you twist from the waist and travels along the arms.

1. Begin with your left hand at eye level and your right directly in front of the lower dan tien at the lowest part of your abdomen.

2. Twist from your waist to the level, left hand held horizontally in front of your face. The right hand travels with the movement of the trunk leading with the inside of the wrist. Fingers should not be stiff and should be held apart so that you can look between your fingers. By allowing the muscles around your waist to relax you will be able to turn much further to each side.

3. Sweep back and forth, changing which hand is on top each time. The important thing to remember is that the movement is gentle and loose, arms sweeping gracefully from side to side.

Repetitions: Eighteen waves sweeping from side to side.

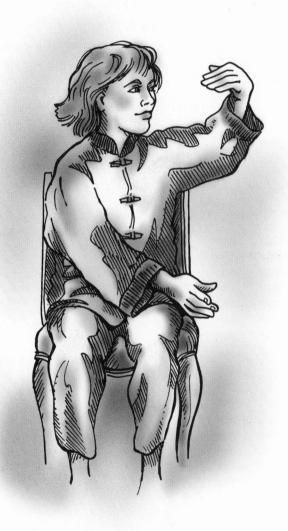

Hands Waving in Clouds

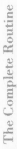

The Complete Routine

Benefits: Loosens and strengthens the shoulders and arms as well as reducing flab at the back of the arm by tightening those muscles.

Posture: Begin by sitting with your back against the back of the chair. Legs should be shoulder-width apart, feet flat on the floor. Tuck your hips under slightly and curve your shoulders inward without hunching. Hold your head lightly on your neck as though it were suspended by a string from the ceiling.

Visualization: Picture yourself holding a light bag and swinging it over your shoulders with no strain. Even though you are not straining, the muscles, particularly at the back of your arms, will become taut and sculpted.

Pathways: Energy moves through the meridians on the outside of your arms, into your hands, and back through the pathway on the inside of your arms.

1. Bring both arms over your right shoulder, muscles very relaxed. Your left hand should be level with your shoulder, your right hand in line with your right ear.

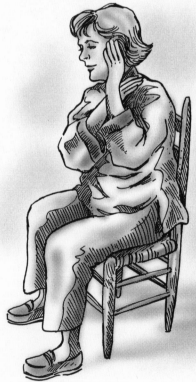

Green Dragon

2. Lower your hands slowly so that the left crosses your chest, brushing your left thigh, ending palm downward to the side of that thigh. Tighten the muscles of your arm as you lower it.

3. The right hand ends in front of the upper chest, held perpendicular to your body so that your palm is facing left. This is the knife-hand position in T'ai Chi. By the time your hand reaches the front of your chest, the muscles of your right arm should be taut.

4. Reverse your original position so that your right hand is almost cupping your left shoulder and your left hand is level with your left ear.

5. Sweep both arms downward again.

6. Your right hand will finish alongside your right thigh and your left in the knife position in front of your chest.

Repetitions: Nine on each side for a total of eighteen dragons.

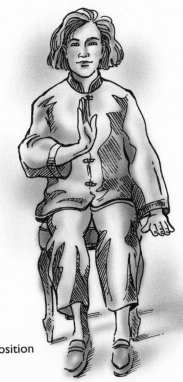

Green Dragon or Knife-Hand Position

❦ Repulse Monkey

Benefits: Repetition of this movement will bring a considerable amount of energy to your hands and will bring your body into balance.

Posture: As in the previous exercise.

Visualization: Imagine the electric currents passing between your hands as you pass one over the other.

Pathways: Both meridians in each of your arms sends the energy into the juncture points on your palms where the localization of that energy can be felt in the waves of vibration between your hands.

1. Hold your left hand at face level with the palm facing upward.
2. Swing your right arm back, following the motion with your eyes by turning your head to look over your shoulder.
3. Now, sweep your arm forward and over your shoulder so that your right hand will pass over your left about 2 to 3 inches above it.
4. Bring your right hand past your left hand facing slightly forward, fingers curled a bit.
5. Turn your right hand palm up, and swing your left arm behind you as you turn your head to follow the motion.
6. Bring the left hand over the right (palms will be facing) without touching your hands together.
7. Slide the left hand forward palm slightly raised, fingers curled.

Repetitions: Nine on each side for a total of eighteen.

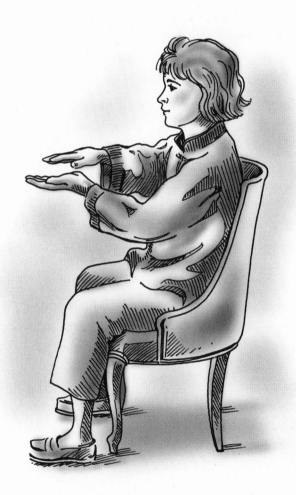

Repulse Monkey

∾ Plucking Thread

Benefits: Again, this exercise tones the arms. Your eye muscles will benefit from following each up and down movement.

Posture: As in the previous exercises.

Visualization: Picture yourself pulling threads out of a piece of cloth, one by one. At the same time, you are pulling the energy from the lower dan tien through the center of your body and up to the level of your eyes.

Pathways: Both the meridians in your arms as well as the pathways in your trunk are being stimulated to release energy to the upper body.

1. Start with your hands resting on your thighs.
2. Curl your right hand to form a bird beak, with all fingers touching your thumb.
3. Breathe in deeply expanding your diaphragm and pluck the thread from between your knees. Raise your arm to the level of your eyes. Follow the movement from knees to face with your eyes.
4. Then, return your hand, wrist leading downward to between your knees as you exhale and tighten your abdomen. Then, raise your arm again and repeat the arm movement and breathing.
   Repetitions: Nine
5. Change hands and repeat the up and down movement. Track the motion of your arm with your eyes. Don't forget to breathe in deeply as you raise your arm and exhale while tightening your abdomen as you lower your arm.
   Repetitions: Nine
6. Using both hands, pluck thread from between your knees, both hands formed in a bird beak Breathe as you did when using one arm at a time.
   Repetitions: Nine

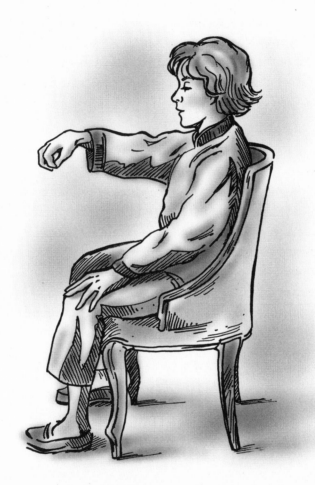

Plucking Thread

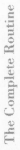

∾ Trunk Rotations

Benefits: This exercise loosens the hip joints, stretches the muscles of the back while reducing your waistline and tightening your abdomen.

Posture: As in the previous exercises.

Visualization: Think about the energy being generated throughout your upper body. Imagine the destruction of fat particles as they are broken up and flushed through your system.

Pathways: All of the upper body is invigorated as energy passes through the meridians at the front, back, center, and waist. Juncture points are opened to release obstructions.

1. Begin again with your hands resting on your thighs.
2. Breathe in deeply, expanding your diaphragm.
3. Circle your trunk to the right, brushing the tops of your thighs with your chest. Blow out your breath and tighten your abdomen.
4. Continue circling to the left side, and return to the center.
5. Take a deep breath again and circle counterclockwise, exhaling as you bend toward your thighs.
   Repetitions: Nine
6. From the center, circle your trunk to the left or clockwise, breathing in before you begin. Exhale as you reach the lowest point of the arc. Then, tighten your abdomen as your chest brushes the tops of your thighs.
   Repetitions: Nine

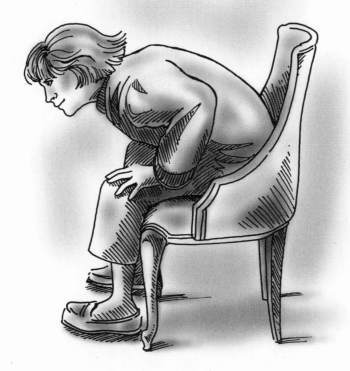

Trunk Rotations

∾ Centering Ch'i

Benefits: Centers the energy and rebalances the body.

Posture: As in the previous exercise.

Visualization: Imagine that you are collecting the ch'i and bits of energy from all over your body returning them to a neutral position at the lower dan tien so that none will be lost or trapped elsewhere in the body.

Pathways: You are targeting all the pathways you have used in the previous exercises.

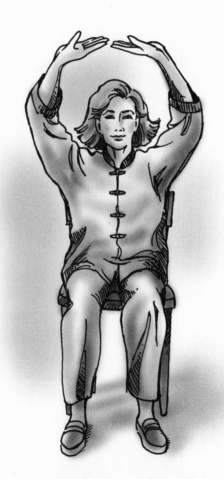

Centering Ch'i

1. Hold your hands palm up just above your lap. Breathe in deeply through your nose while contracting your diaphragm. In this exercise, the diaphragm is not expanded during inhalations.

2. As you tighten your diaphragm and abdomen, raise your arms out to the side and up over your head to its center. Your palms are now facing the ceiling, fingers barely touching.

3. Allow your arms to descend gradually in an arc out to the side. As you do so, exhale until there is no breath left in your lungs and relax the muscles of your diaphragm and abdomen.

4. Return your arms to the original position in front of the lowest part of your abdomen, palms facing upward.

Repetitions: Three

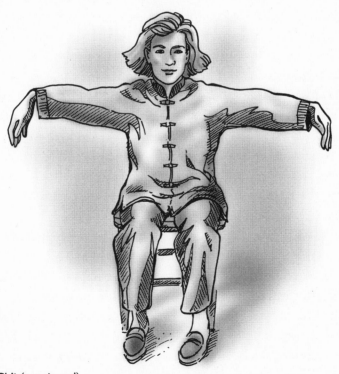

Centering Ch'i (continued)

Lower-Body Exercises

Despite the fact that there are certain limitations in performing lower-body exercises sitting down, you can achieve remarkable results. Seated T'ai Chi offers all the stretching and strengthening exercises that are available in standing programs. Also, doing T'ai Chi in a chair does not limit the exercise's special emphasis on the spatial relationship between our bodies and our environment. The emphasis on deep, diaphragmatic breathing and the involvement of the mind in accessing the energy that is natural in all humans sets this program apart from the more familiar exercise routines.

We begin our lower-body exercises in another burst of oxygen with a deep breath and expansion of the diaphragm as our arms are raised overhead. We roll up on the balls of the feet while envisioning the sparks of energy from the lower dan tien coursing through thighs, lower legs and feet. We are moving energy through the yangqiaomei, into the yongquan (the juncture point on the sole of the foot). As you press your arms palm down alongside your thighs, pull your feet back on to the heels. In this movement, we are returning the energy back up the inside of the leg via the yinqiaomei, through the huiyin and back to the lower dan tien. We are following the usual rule again here: inhale deeply when your arms are raised and exhale as your arms are lowered. To loosen ankle joints, we roll back and forth from the balls of the feet to the heels in a very relaxed way. Then we lift our feet off the floor and point and flex alternately followed by circling one foot at a time, clockwise and counterclockwise. None of these movements should be forced.

When you roll up on the ball of the foot again (one foot at a time), you will be using the resistance of the floor to strengthen your arch, breathing into the forward roll, and breathing out when the foot is rocked back on to the heel. Hold each position for fifteen to thirty seconds. This exercise works not only the ankle but also the calf when your foot is rolled up on to the ball and the Achilles' tendon when you have pulled back on your heel.

The purpose for the last of the foot and ankle exercises is to once again relax the muscles and tendons in this area. This section begins with your leg out to the side of the chair, foot poised on the big toe. As you circle first clockwise and then counterclockwise, breathe into the movement and imagine that you have rag doll ankles—loose, loose, loose. Above all, don't tense the leg and ankle muscles trying to make a perfect circle with your heel. The same admonition applies to shaking out your feet. My elderly students refer to this exercise as "jello feet" and that is exactly how it should be performed.

After the foot and ankle exercises, we'll go to work on the knees. Your feet will be together and flat on the floor. You'll need to scoot forward on your chair so you'll have more leverage. Obviously, circling your knees will be more difficult since you're seated. The secret here, again, is to relax the muscles and joints of the legs, ankles, and knees until you can approximate a circular motion. Using your hands you will then push your knees apart as far as they can go with your feet still flat on the floor. Allow the knees to fall back together naturally. Don't use too much force when pushing the knees apart: we'll be getting a good inner-thigh stretch in the next exercise.

With your back once more against the back of the chair, begin the chair straddle by moving one leg at a time out to the side as far as it will go, followed by the other. Hold for a second or two and then return your legs to the front of the chair. Continue straddling the chair, moving one leg at a time out to the side and alternate legs each time.

For the next exercise you will need to angle yourself on the chair. Stretch one leg to the side and back while keeping your foot flat on the floor. To do that, you will have to release your ankle to allow it to bend over the inside of the foot. One way to ensure that your foot remains flat is to slide your leg backwards rather than placing it behind you. Turn to the other side, legs together, and repeat alternately from leg to leg.

Golden Cockerel is a challenge for your sense of balance when practiced standing. Since we are seated, balance won't be the issue, but there will be a certain amount of pressure on the hip joint and the muscles on the top of the thigh. From the knee down, your leg is completely relaxed and your toe should be pointed downward. Use your stomach muscles to take some of the pressure off your hip and thigh. This is a good exercise to strengthen your thigh muscles and your abdomen as well.

Because your leg must be held straight out to the front as you perform the Needle at the Bottom of the Sea exercise, all the muscles of your legs will be getting a good workout. Stretching the opposite hand until at least your fingers reach the floor will lengthen the muscles of your back and buttocks as well as those of your shoulder and arm. Breathing out as you stretch your arm toward the floor will help. Alternate arms and legs each time, making certain that you do an equal number on each side.

Leg Sweeps Lotus will stretch and relax your leg muscles while at the same time stimulating the glands in the groin area that are part of the immune system. These glands belong to the lymphatic system that seeks out and destroys harmful bacteria and other foreign agents. Swinging one leg over the other activates the lymph nodes in this area producing more disease-fighting lymph.

As usual, Centering Ch'i concludes this section of the exercises. The return of ch'i to its proper location prepares you for the last and final portion of the seated T'ai Chi program: relaxation and self-massage.

Lower-Body Exercises

∾ Loosening Knees

Benefits: The knee joints may have become tense during the last exercise. Now, we are going to relax and loosen the knees.

Posture: Sit forward on your chair feet and knees together. Bend over slightly from the hips and place your hands on your knees, cupping the joints.

Visualization: Imagine your knees as loose and pliable, the synovial fluid around the kneecap as flowing freely, nourishing and lubricating the moving surfaces of the joint.

Pathways: Yangqiaomei, the outer meridian of the leg joins with the yinqiaomei at the laogong point on the sole of your foot just behind the ball. Together they release energy to heal and strengthen the knee joint.

1. With your hands, rotate your knees to the right or clockwise. Try not to move your body any more than is absolutely necessary. Isolate your arms and legs by relaxing your hip and shoulder muscles so that your whole body is not rotating.
   Repetitions: Nine

2. Reverse the direction so that you are now circling your knees to the left or counterclockwise.

Repetitions: Nine

3. Now, push your knees gently apart while keeping your feet together. Allow your knees to close back together.

Repetitions: Nine

∾ Chair Straddles

Benefits: This exercise stretches and strengthens the inner thigh replacing flab with muscle.

Posture: Begin by sitting with your back against the back of the chair. Legs should be shoulder-width apart, feet flat on the floor. Tuck your hips under slightly and curve your shoulders inward without hunching. Hold your head lightly on your neck as though it were suspended by a string from the ceiling.

Visualization: Imagine that you can see through your skin to the thigh muscles underneath. See the muscles as they lengthen and contract, breaking up the fat particles and tightening the skin.

Pathways: Energy is released through the meridian on the outside of your legs, through the sole of your foot and back up the meridian on the inside of your legs.

1. Breathe in, expanding your diaphragm as you slide your right leg first, then your left leg out to the side of your chair.

2. Blow out your breath as you press both legs back as far as you can. Releasing your breath will relax the muscles allowing for a wider stretch. Breathe normally as you hold the straddle position for ten seconds.

3. Continue alternating the lead leg, pressing and holding the straddle for ten seconds each time.

Repetitions: Eighteen

Pushing Up Sky with Foot Rolls

Benefits: This exercise stretches the whole body while strengthening the feet and loosening the ankle joints.

Posture: Begin by sitting with your back against the back of the chair. Legs should be shoulder-width apart, feet flat on the floor. Tuck your hips under slightly and curve your shoulders inward without hunching. Hold your head lightly on your neck as though it were suspended by a string from the ceiling.

Visualization: Imagine that you are exchanging energy with the sky as you push up toward the ceiling and with the earth as you press the balls of your feet firmly on the floor.

Pathways: All meridians of the body are utilized in this exercise but, most particularly, the two meridians in the arms and the two in the legs.

1. Roll your feet up on to the balls of your feet while at the same time pressing your arms toward the ceiling, palms up.

2. Take a deep breath as you lift your arms and roll your feet, expanding your diaphragm but keeping your back against the back of the chair.

3. Now, bring your arms down alongside your thighs, palms toward the floor while simultaneously, rolling your feet back on to the heels.

4. Breathe out and tighten your abdomen as you change the position of your arms and feet.

   Repetitions: Nine

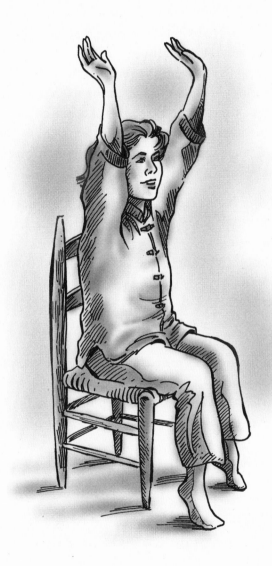

Pushing Up Sky with Foot Rolls

～ Ankle Presses and Circles

Benefits: This exercise first loosens your ankle joints in a relaxed way. With your feet off the floor, your thigh muscles are tightened, stretched, and toned. Ankle presses strengthen your feet and ankles.

Posture: As in the previous exercise.

Visualization: Imagine your ankles are soft and rubbery during the relaxed exercises. During the pressing and lifting exercises, picture the strength and tautness of your thigh, feet, and ankle muscles.

Pathways: The meridians receiving the most stimulation are the two that run up and down your legs. The juncture point on the bottom of your foot is being cleared of any obstructions.

1. Begin with your hands resting comfortably on your thighs.
2. Rock your feet back and forth from the heels to the balls without tension.
   Repetitions: Nine
3. Lift your feet off the floor, thighs straight out in front of you. Flex and point your toes.
   Repetitions: Nine
4. Now, circle one foot at a time, to the inside. Reverse, and circle one foot at a time to the outside.
   Repetitions: Nine circles for each direction with each foot for a total of thirty-six individual circles.
5. Return your feet to the floor. Press up firmly on the ball of your right foot. Hold for a moment and then rock back on your heel and hold again.
   Repetitions: Nine
6. Change to your left foot and repeat the sequence of ball and hold and heel and hold.
   Repetitions: Nine
7. Slide your right leg over the side of the chair. Balance on the big toe and circle your heel in one direction then in the other.
   Repetitions: Nine in each direction for a total of eighteen circles.

8. Slide your left foot out to the side of your chair and repeat the sequence of inside and outside circles using your big toe as the pivot.

Repetitions: Nine in each direction for a total of eighteen individual circles.

9. Lift your feet off the floor, legs straight in front of you, and wag your feet for about ten seconds to loosen the ankle joint.

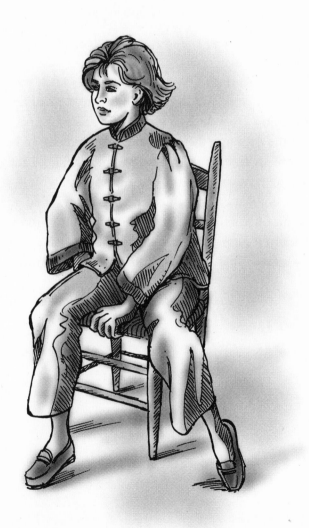

Ankle Circles

∾ Bow Stance

Benefits: This is a total leg stretch beginning at the hip and is intended to trim and tone the leg muscles.

Posture: As in the previous exercise.

Visualization: Once again, imagine the fat particles as they break apart and flush away. Feel your thigh muscles as they become stronger and more taut.

Pathway: Energy is again set loose to invigorate the muscles of the legs through the meridians on the outside and inside of the leg.

1. Turn to your left so that you are angled on your chair. Keep your legs together.

2. Breathe in deeply and then exhale as you stretch your right leg out to the side of your chair and as far behind you as possible. Keep your foot flat on the floor. To make this movement easier at first, start with your foot flat on the floor and then, slide it along the floor and extend your leg until your knee is straight. Breathe normally and hold for ten seconds.

3. Now, angle yourself on the chair to the right. Slide your left foot out to the side and back until your knee is straight. Hold again for ten seconds.

4. Continue alternating sides/legs, keeping your working leg stretched to the maximum for a period of ten seconds each time.

   Repetitions: Nine stretches with each leg for a total of eighteen.

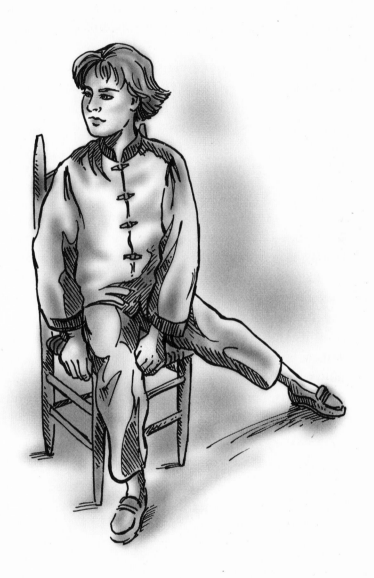

Bow Stance

Benefits: Like the previous exercises, repetition of this movement trims and tones the leg muscles particularly those of the thigh. Since the abdominal muscles are used in the leg lifts, the abdomen itself is firmed and the belly reduced.

Posture: As in the previous exercises.

Visualization: Imagine a string attached to the base of your rib cage, intertwined through the abdominal muscles and attached to the tops of your thighs. As you lift your rib cage and tighten your abdomen, your thigh is pulled upward toward your torso.

Pathways: Energy travels through the four meridians in the trunk and the two in the legs involving the middle and lower dan tiens.

1. Breathe in as you lift your rib cage and tighten your abdomen. At the same time, lift your right leg, knee bent, as high as possible.

2. Hold your working leg in position for the duration of the inward breath and then, lower your leg slowly as you release your breath and relax your abdomen. Be aware that the breathing pattern here is *reverse* breathing like that used in Centering Ch'i.

3. Now, breathe in deeply and as you lift your rib cage and tighten your abdomen, lift your left leg, and hold. Exhale gradually and lower your leg slowly.

Repetitions: Nine lifts with each leg for a total of eighteen.

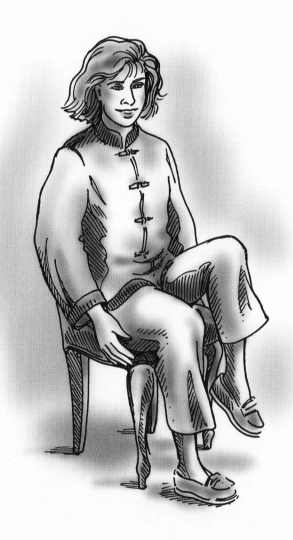

Golden Cockerel Stands on One Leg

Benefits: This exercise is a wonderful stretch of the back muscles and helps to trim and tone the legs.

Posture: As in the previous exercises.

Visualization: Imagine the energy circulating from the top of your head to the bottom of your feet. Think of the fat particles breaking apart and being flushed through your system.

Pathways: Energy is traveling through all of the meridians, invigorating, and warming the whole body.

1. Inhale deeply while in your beginning posture.
2. Lift your right leg with the knee straight.
3. Blow out your breath to relax your muscles as you bend from your hips and reach with your left hand between your legs to the floor.
4. Lift your left leg, keeping your knee straight, and reach to the floor with your right hand as you exhale slowly and in time with your bending motion.

   Repetitions: Eighteen floor touches.

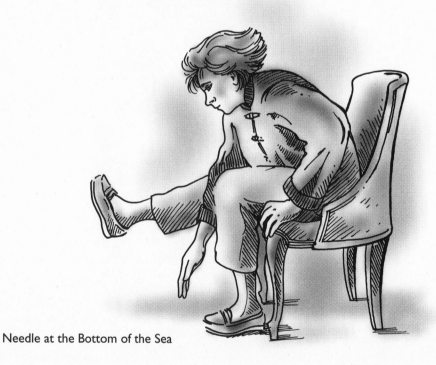

Needle at the Bottom of the Sea

∽ Leg Sweeps Lotus

Benefits: This exercise stimulates the lymph glands located in the groin. The movements limber up the hips, reducing daily stress on this weight-bearing joint as well as strengthening the joint to prevent injury.

Posture: As in the previous exercises.

Visualization: Picture the energy moving in and around the hip joint and through the groin. Imagine the increased production of lymphocytes.

Pathways: The lower dan tien releases energy to the hip and groin through the four meridians in the torso and the two leg meridians.

1. Sweep your right leg up and across your left thigh. Return to the beginning position so that your right leg is in line with your right shoulder.

2. Lift the left leg and swing it across your right thigh. Return to the usual position.

3. Continue alternating, brushing one leg as far across the other as possible. Your working leg may be straight or slightly bent to allow you to cross over further.

Repetitions: Nine sweeps with each leg for a total of eighteen.

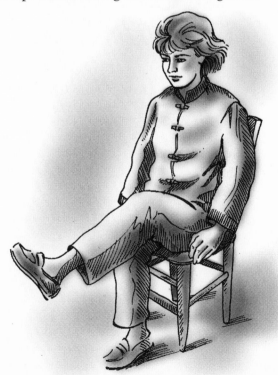

Leg Sweeps Lotus

⌇ Centering Ch'i

Benefits: Centers the energy and rebalances the body.

Posture: As in the previous exercise.

Visualization: Imagine that you are collecting the ch'i and bits of energy from all over your body returning them to a neutral position at the lower dan tien so that none will be lost or trapped elsewhere in the body.

Pathways: You are targeting all the pathways you have used in the previous exercises.

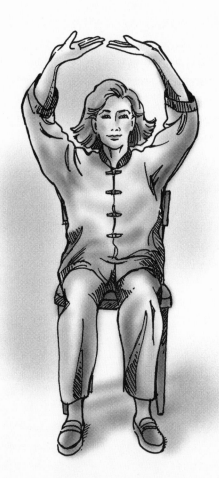

Centering Ch'i

1. Hold your hands palm up just above your lap. Breathe in deeply through your nose while contracting your diaphragm. In this exercise, the diaphragm is **not** expanded during inhalations.

2. As you tighten your diaphragm and abdomen, raise your arms out to the side and up over your head to its center. Your palms are now facing the ceiling, fingers barely touching.

3. Allow your arms to descend gradually in an arc out to the side. As you do so, exhale until there is no breath left in your lungs and relax the muscles of your diaphragm and abdomen.

4. Return your arms to the original position in front of the lowest part of your abdomen, palms facing upward.

   Repetitions: Three.

   Relax for a moment before beginning the next set of exercises.

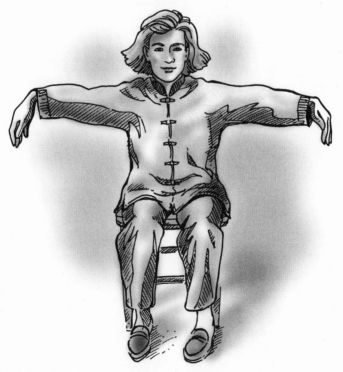

Centering Ch'i (continued)

One of my favorite poems was written by Deng Ming-Dao in which the author describes a cat sitting in the sun, a turtle sitting on a rock lifting her head upward to the sun, and a frog seated on a lily pad. The question the author asks is "why aren't people so smart?" Why do we consider quiet time to be such an unimportant or, worse, a "peculiar" practice? Meditative stillness need not be associated with a particular religious belief. It should not be considered a burden nor a task to be discharged when we would rather be doing something else. Like dogs and cats and frogs and turtles, we too need a time of stillness, every bit as much as we need the air we breathe and the food we eat. If we accept the Taoist belief that the universe is a seamless web, a totality of existence where no thing and no one stands alone, then we must be open to receive the lessons nature teaches us. Whether we look to agriculture as the early Taoists did, to our own gardens or to the animals that inhabit our homes, we see a pattern of life that we would do well to imitate. Why can't we be like the dog lying in the grass, the turtle stretching its neck to receive the warmth of the sun's rays, or the frog resting peacefully on the lily pad?

In this portion of seated T'ai Chi, we will strive for peace of mind and soul, and a total relaxation of the body. Here, we will recharge our batteries; recenter our energy; and rebalance our whole selves, mind, body, and spirit. For a few moments, at least, we will experience what it means to just be.

Acupressure and Self-Massage

All exercise classes end with a cool-down session of some kind. Seated T'ai Chi concludes with acupressure and self-massage. The acupressure points in this section are by no means the only points available for your use. They are simply the ones I've found to be the most popular. If you have health challenges not covered by the points in the following Relaxation section, consult Chapter 5 for a complete listing and explanation of many more acupressure points that may be of benefit to you.

In acupressure, the only equipment required is your own fingers and hands. Through acupressure and self-massage you can be proactive with your own health. For many common, everyday aches, pains, and ailments you will be able to rely on yourself to relieve the symptoms and rebalance your body. You can use acupressure on yourself or others safely and repetitively. This form of therapy requires no particular training other than experimentation by you to determine which points will be the most useful for your needs. With a little practice you will become adept at finding the exact spots on your skin that you are looking for and will learn how much pressure is appropriate in each case.

The regular use of these pressure points has a number of health benefits. Many of the following points, as well as those in Chapter 5, stimulate the immune system to prevent diseases that are acquired simply by breathing the air or by coming in contact with someone who is carrying a virus. Acupressure will balance the internal environment of your body and counterbalance your body to adjust to changes in your immediate surroundings. In addition, frequent use of the proper acupressure points will reduce tension and increase circulation.

There are points that have been in use for many centuries to treat ailments and relieve aches and pains by blocking the pain gates, or neurochemicals, of the brain. Pressing on particular points allows the ch'i or energy to flow unimpeded through the meridians and systems of you body. Stimulating blood and lymph flow makes you more resistant to disease and can aid in weight loss by balancing the digestive system and reducing the stress that sometimes contributes to overeating and weight gain.

The Benefits of Massage

Self-massage, though not quite as relaxing as massage therapy performed by someone else, is an efficient way to reduce tension and stress without the time and expense necessary for a visit to a professional therapist. Massage, much like acupressure, stimulates the flow of blood and lymph to all parts of the body. Massage also stimulates the nerve receptors on the skin. The movement of your hands over your arms, shoulders, face, and legs will cause the blood vessels to dilate, thereby facilitating the flow of blood. Pressing against your skin reaches the muscles underneath causing the muscles to expand and contract and assisting the circulation of lymph. The gentle stretching action of the muscles during a massage keeps the surrounding tissues elastic making them more supportive and less inclined to injury during physical activity.

Oxygen capacity can increase after massage by as much as 10 to 15 percent. The body's secretions and excretions are also increased by massage along with a boost to the metabolic rate. When the metabolic rate increases, the body's cells absorb and utilize the fuel provided by food at a faster rate which, in turn, reduces the absorption and storage of fat. By rubbing along the surface of your skin, you are stimulating the nerve endings, which increases the flow of nourishing blood to your internal organs.

Regular massage enhances the condition of the skin by stimulating the oil and sweat glands. Increasing the production of sweat clears toxins from the body and the surface of the skin. The additional output of oils from the sebaceous glands lubricates and softens the skin.

Eighty percent of all diseases are stress related. Frustration, insecurity, and stress cause the overproduction by the adrenal gland of the hormones norepinephrine and hydrocortisone. Too much norepinephrine and hydrocortisone constrict the blood vessels (vasoconstriction) reducing the flow of blood through the veins and arteries. This constriction makes the heart work harder, breathing more rapid and shallow, and slows the digestive processes. The result can be migraines, hypertension, depression, or indigestion. Massage, along with the appropriate acupressure points, reduces stress, increases circulation, facilitates digestion, and opens the chest cavity and lungs for deeper, more healthful breathing.

∾ Face and Head

You will be using three acupressure points in this first section. They are the Third Eye Point, the Posterior Summit, and the Wind Mansion Point. As you press on the Third Eye Point, think back to the Needle at the Bottom of the Sea exercise in the previous section of lower-body stretches. The needle represents the elusive fount of creativity in all of us. While you are pressing on the Third Eye Point, concentrate on moving the creativity upwards and into this point. The Posterior Summit relaxes you while it clears the brain of psychological conflicts or trauma. The Wind Mansion Point will relieve tension from the head and neck.

Benefits: Relaxes all muscles that may have become stressed during the previous exercises and returns body, mind, and spirit to a state of calm.

Posture: Begin by sitting with your back against the back of the chair. Legs should be shoulder-width apart, feet flat on the floor. Tuck your hips under slightly and curve your shoulders inward without hunching. Hold your head lightly on your neck as though it were suspended by a string from the ceiling.

Visualization: Picture the energy moving through your body bringing calm to your mind and emotions.

Pathways: The meridian that travels up your spine ends at the upper palate behind your teeth. The pathway that runs down the front of your body, begins on the tip of the tongue. The chongmei governs the center of the body connecting the three dan tiens. All of these are being both stimulated and soothed.

Acupressure Points: GV 24.5, GV 19, and GV 16

1. Rub your palms briskly together until they are warm. Close your eyes and place your warm palms over them. Hold for about thirty seconds.

2. Then, steeple your hands and press against the Third Eye Point (see page 94) that is above your nose bone and between your eyebrows. If you are congested due to allergies or a cold, use the middle finger of your left hand to press the Third Eye Point and the middle finger of your right hand to press on the top of your head where a baby's soft spot is (the Posterior Summit point). Hold for thirty seconds.

3. Pinch your eyebrows gently between your thumb and index fingers. Beginning at the inside corner, slide your fingers along your brows to the outside corners. Keep your eyes closed while you concentrate on relaxing your eye muscles.
   Repetitions: Nine

4. Massage your temples with your fingertips, upward and outward.
   Repetitions: Nine

5. Massage from the base of your nose along the cheekbone to the outside

edge or your eyes. If your sinuses are congested, you will feel immediate relief as you run your fingertips along the side of your nose.

Repetitions: Nine

6. Using your fingertips again, massage from the base of your jaw on either side of your mouth upward and outward. Don't bear down too hard, but exert enough pressure to bring the healing blood to the surface of your skin.

   Repetitions: Nine

7. The Chinese believe that all parts of the body including organs, joints, skeletal structure, and so on are represented on the ear. Give your ears a thorough going over as though your were washing them.

   Repetitions: Nine

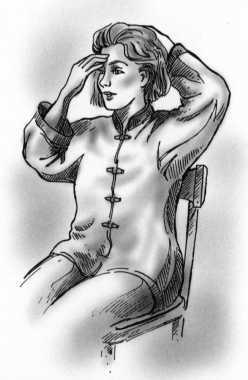

Third Eye Point with the Posterior Summit Point

8. Using both thumbs (if you don't have a hearing aid) rub along the mastoid process at the back of the ears.

9. Press your middle finger at the base of the skull, in the area of the basal ganglia. This is the pressure point called the Wind Mansion. Hold your finger there for twenty to thirty seconds.

10. Then, begin tapping with the fingertips of both hands up from the base of the skull just above the Wind Mansion (the basal ganglia) through the center of the head (hands close together). When you reach the hairline, using one hand on each side tap along the sides of the head in the general shape of the right and left hemispheres of the brain. Tapping the head with the fingertips is thought to stimulate the brain and improve memory.
   Repetitions: Nine

11. Press with the heel of your hand on the frontal bones. Move your hands to the side of your head and press on the temporal bones on each side. Move your hands back further and toward the top of your head and press against the bones covering the parietal lobe. At the back of your head just above the ridge at the base of the skull is the occipital bone. Press in this area with your finger tips for a few seconds.

12. Relax your arms while you circle your tongue, mouth closed, clockwise and then, counterclockwise.
    Repetitions: Nine

13. Press—don't grind—your front teeth together. Work your jaw muscle strongly by pressing the back teeth together on one side. Change sides and repeat. Press your front teeth together again.
    Repetitions: Nine times for each section of teeth.

14. Clasp your hands together behind your head. Push against your hands using your neck muscles.
    Bring your hands down to your thighs and rest.
    Repetitions: Nine push/release movements.

There are many pressure points that are effective for relieving headaches, sinus pressure or tired and irritated eyes. However, it is best to use the points described in the preceding exercises for at least one month. In that time, you will become familiar with the location of each point and the amount of pressure that is most comfortable and healing for you. After you become accustomed to using acupressure, you may want to experiment with the additional pressure points for the head, face, and neck.

Turn to Chapter 5 for the location and benefits of each of the following points:

* Drilling Bamboo—B 2 (see pages 184, 204, 207, 211)
* Facial Beauty—St 3 (see pages 184, 205, 207)
* Four Whites—St 2 (see page 205)
* Heavenly Pillar—B 10 (see pages 188, 211)
* Jaw Chariot—St 6 (see page 208)
* Listening Place—SI 19 (see pages 204, 208)
* Ear Gate—TW 21 (see pages 204, 208)
* Reunion of Hearing—GB 2 (see pages 204, 208)
* Windscreen—TW 17 (see pages 204, 209)
* Window of Heaven—TW 16 (see page 212)

Diagrams of the location of these points can be found in Appendix A.

∾ Thymus

The thymus is located in a small depression directly below the V of your collarbone. It is a mass of glandular tissue related to the endocrine system and the first gland to develop in the fetus. It is responsible for the later and continuing development of the entire immune system. The thymus gland processes white blood cells or lymphocytes These lymphocytes seek out and destroy foreign substances that may grow within or invade the body from without. The thymus continues to grow throughout childhood and puberty but gradually decreases in size as we mature.

Benefits: Considered the youth gland in ancient China, this area was stimulated to ward off illness and to keep the body vigorous and youthful.

Posture: Begin by sitting with your back against the back of the chair. Legs should be shoulder-width apart, feet flat on the floor. Tuck your hips under slightly and curve your shoulders inward without hunching. Hold your head lightly on your neck as though it were suspended by a string from the ceiling.

Visualization: As you massage the thymus, imagine that you are releasing immune-producing energy throughout your entire body destroying harmful bacteria and the free radicals that cause aging.

Pathways: By stimulating the thymus gland, energy is freed to travel along the meridian that runs down the center of your body, the daimei that circles your waist, as well as the pathway up your spine and the center chongmei connecting all the ch'i points together.

1. Run your finger along your collarbone until you locate the V directly above the breastbone.
2. Half a finger width below that V you will feel a small depression. The thymus gland is behind the hollow.
3. Press your index or middle finger firmly on this spot and hold for at least thirty seconds. You may also circle your finger on the indentation clockwise for the same amount of time.

∽ Shoulders and Arms

Benefits: Much of our daily stress results in pain and tension in the shoulders. The warmth and motion of your hands will reduce that feeling and give you a burst of energy. The motion of your hands as they massage up and down, will bring fresh blood to the surface of the skin firming and toning your arms.

Posture: As in the previous exercise.

Visualization: Picture a soothing spray of warm water pouring over your shoulders and down your arms relaxing all the muscles.

Pathways: By massaging from the shoulders and down through your arms you will be stimulating the flow of energy through the meridian on the outside of your arms, through the middle fingers and back up the inside pathway. Pause at the juncture point on your palm to break up any obstructions that may have accumulated at that point.

Acupressure Points: LI 11, LI 4, GB 21, and H 7

1. With your opposite hand, brush your fingers from back to front over your shoulder.
   Repetitions: Nine

2. At the highest point on the shoulder muscle approximately half of the distance from the spine to the outer edge of the shoulder is the pressure point called the Shoulder Well. Press firmly with your middle finger on this point for thirty seconds.

3. On the same side, run your fingertips along the outside of your arm, over the middle finger and to the juncture point on your palm where you should pause and press for a moment. To find this point, curl your fingers into a fist. Where the middle finger meets the palm is the laogong, or junction of the two pathways that bring energy into your arms.

4. Continue with your fingertips from the juncture point back up the inside of your arms to your shoulder.
   Repetitions: Nine strokes down the outside of your arm and back up the inside.

5. Change sides and repeat the massaging motions first on the shoulder and then down the outside of the arm and back up the inside. Return to the middle of the muscle on the top of the shoulder midway between the spine and the furthest end of the shoulder (the Shoulder Well). Press with the middle finger of your opposite arm and hold for thirty seconds to relieve feelings of irritability and frustration. Breathe deeply as you press on this point.
   Repetitions: Nine

6. Cross your arms and find the end of the elbow crease on the top of each arm. This point is called the Crooked Pond. This pressure point may be used to stimulate you immune system. It is also effective for relieving constipation, the fever of a cold, and arthritic pain in the elbow.

7. Press with your index or middle finger on the opposite elbow and hold for at least thirty seconds. Breathe deeply in through your nose and out through your mouth, expanding and contracting your diaphragm with each breath.

8. Press the flap of skin between your index finger and your thumb just in front of the joint between the two fingers with the index finger and thumb of your opposite hand. This is the Joining the Valley point and is very helpful for increasing your immunity, cleansing your liver, or reducing feelings of depression. Hold for thirty seconds and then change hands.

9. Now, use a washing motion to massage your hands, back, palm, and fingers. Continue for a few moments until your hands are thoroughly warmed.

10. Using your opposite hand, press the blood to the fingertips by massaging upward on each finger. Then, change hands and repeat for each finger.
    Repetitions: Three upward motions on each finger.

11. Turn your wrist (either arm) so that the inside of the wrist is facing you. Run your finger along the wrist crease until you come to the end of it at the base of the little finger. This is the location of the Spirit Gate pressure point. Use of this point will relieve anxiety and insomnia. Press and hold for at least thirty seconds as you breathe deeply.

12. Play the vertical flute by placing your left hand at the level of your abdomen and your right hand directly above it. Beginning with the little finger of your left hand, separate each finger, curling and uncurling as though you were pressing on the openings on a flute.

13. When you reach the top finger, which will be the thumb of your right hand, reverse the motion moving back down the length of your flute.
    Repetitions: Three runs up and down the flute.

14. Change hands so that the right is now on the bottom and the left on top.

Repeat the curling and uncurling of the fingers from hand to hand and back again.

Repetitions: Three runs again up and down the flute.

If you are still experiencing tension or pain in your arms and shoulders after a month of using the acupressure points described in the preceding exercises, you may want to experiment with one or two of the other healing points for this part of the body. Turn to Chapter 5 for a description of the all the benefits and the location of the following additional acupressure points.

* Gates of Consciousness—GB 20 (see pages 187, 196, 211, 227)
* Heavenly Rejuvenation—TW 15 (see pages 194, 230)
* Outer Arm Bone—LI 14 (see page 230)
* Active Pond—TW 4 (see Appendix A)
* Big Mound—P 7 (see Appendix A)
* Inner Gate—P 6 (see pages 195, 197, 229)

Diagrams of the location of these points can be found in Appendix A.

ᔇ Abdomen, Hips, and Lower Back

Benefits: Relieves bloating as well as both constipation and diarrhea. The brushing movement soothes and tightens the abdominal muscles for a firmer, flatter stomach. Using a circular motion for the hips warms the joints by increasing the circulation to that area. The warmth of your hands combined with a firm pressure will alleviate the tension that accumulates in the lower back.

Posture: Begin by sitting with your back against the back of the chair. Legs should be shoulder-width apart, feet flat on the floor. Tuck your hips under slightly and curve your shoulders inward without hunching. Hold your head lightly on your neck as though it were suspended by a string from the ceiling.

Visualization: Imagine energy passing around and through the intestines, circling around the hip joints, and sending waves of soothing energy through the lower back.

Pathways: The meridians that travel down the front of the body and the pathway in the center of the body release a soothing energy to the abdomen. The meridian that travels up the back is stimulated to send a stream of energy to the lower back and the hips.

Acupressure Points: B 23, B 47, B 48, and CV 6

1. Hold one hand over the other at waist level. Brush downward with a firm pressure to about three finger widths below the navel.
   Repetitions: Nine

2. Measure two finger widths directly below your navel. Press firmly and hold for thirty seconds to tone weak abdominal muscles, strengthen your back, and alleviate back pain.

3. Use both hands in a circular motion around your right hip moving from back to front (see page 102).
   Repetitions: Nine

4. Change sides and repeat the circling of both hands moving from back to front. Use a firm pressure to stimulate circulation.
   Repetitions: Nine

5. Sit forward on your chair. Place both hands on your lower back. Run your fingertips up and down your back. If you have a backache, circle your hands using the heels of your palms for a deeper massage.
   Repetitions: At least nine presses and nine circles as well, if needed.

6. B 23 and B 47 (the Sea of Vitality points) are in line with each other on your back between the second and third lumbar vertebrae. B 23 (is two finger widths from your spine on either side of the spin. B 47 is four finger widths from the spine on either side. Because these may be awkward spots to reach, locate the areas with your fingers then fist your hands at those spots and lean back against the back of your chair. Continue to lean back against your fists as they are pressed against these two spots for at least thirty to sixty seconds.

7. Find the large bony area at the base of your spine. Measure one to two finger widths from the spine to find the Womb and Vitals acupressure point. Because of the location of these points, fist your hands and lean back into the back of your chair. Hold for thirty seconds while you breathe deeply.

After you have familiarized yourself with the pressure points described in the exercises for the abdomen, hips, and lower back, you may want to incorporate into your daily routine one or two of the additional healing points from the following list. Turn to Chapter 5 for the location and benefits of the following acupressure points for the lower back and hips:

* Crooked Pond—LI 11 (see pages 185, 191, 196, 200)
* Joining the Valley—LI 4 (see pages 186, 192, 200, 208, 216)
* Center of Power—CV 12 (see page 214)

Do not use this point if you have a chronic or life-threatening disease

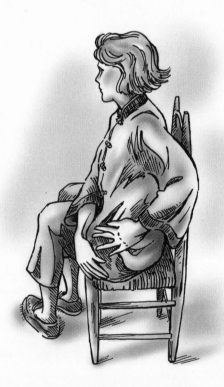

Hip Massage

such as high blood pressure, cancer, or heart disease. Use this point only if you have not eaten in the past couple of hours.

- Gate Origin—CV 4 (see page 222)
- Grandfather Grandson—Sp 4 (see pages 215, 222)
- Rushing Door and Mansion Cottage—Sp 12 and Sp 13 (see page 223)
- Sacral Points—B 27 and B 34 (see page 223)
- Three Yin Crossing—Sp 6 (see pages 223, 225)

Diagrams of the location of these points can be found in Appendix A.

∾ Legs and Knees

Benefits: This exercise stimulates the circulation in your legs, relieving muscle aches. Massaging around the kneecaps promotes the production of synovial fluid for increased flexibility. The acupressure point on the outside of your leg benefits digestion and reduces fatigue. The pressure point at the back of the knee strengthens the lower back and knees.

Posture: As in the previous exercise.

Visualization: Picture the increased flow of blood and energy through the legs and around the knees.

Pathways: You will be running your fingertips along the outside of your leg where the yangqiaomei meridian is located and returning the energy with your fingertips back to the trunk through the yinqiaomei on the inside of the leg.

Acupressure Points: St 36, B 54, and K 6

1. Using the fingertips of your right hand, follow the meridian on the outside of your leg to the top of your foot. Using both hands circle your ankle joint. Then, run your fingertips up the inside of your leg to just below the top of your thigh.

   Repetitions: Nine

2. Now, using the fingertips of your left hand, trace the meridian along the

outside of your left leg to the top of the foot. Circle your left hand around your ankle joint and pick up from the back of the ankle with your right hand, returning by way of the inside pathway up your leg and back to your thigh.

Repetitions: Nine

3. Measure four finger widths below your knee on the outside of the leg. You will find a good-sized depression there. This is the pressure point called the Three Mile Point. This is a particularly effective point for the relief of bloating, cramps, nausea, and indigestion. Press firmly with your middle fingers (one on each leg) and hold for thirty seconds.

4. Press both thumbs in the middle of the creases at the back of your knees. This is the location of the acupressure point called the Commanding Middle. If you have a backache, knee pain or stiffness, arthritis of the knee, or suffer from sciatica, this is a pressure point that you will want to use regularly. Press strongly and hold for at least thirty seconds.

5. Trace with your finger to the bone on the inside of your ankle. Next to the bone is a small indentation. This is the pressure point called Joyful Sleep. It is, as its name implies an effective point to relieve insomnia. Press firmly on this point and hold for at least thirty seconds. Use of this point before bedtime will ensure a good night's sleep.

6. Chronic back pain may be at the root of some sleeping problems so we will use the Calm Sleep point before ending this section. Transfer your hand to the outside of your ankle. Slide your finger down the large ankle bone until you find the first, small indentation. Press firmly on this point with your middle finger and hold for at least thirty seconds. This is another effective point to use at night before you go to bed.

Again, turn to Chapter 5 to find the location and read about the benefits of the following acupressure points you may wish to add or substitute for relief of pain in the lower back, knees, feet or abdomen:

- Calf's Nose—St 35 (see page 219)
- Commanding Activity—B 53 (see page 220)

- Crooked Spring—Lv 8 (see page 220)
- Nourishing Valley—K 10 (see page 220)
- Shady Side of the Mountain—Sp 9 (see pages 220, 225)
- Bigger Stream—K 3 (see pages 203, 218)
- Blazing Valley—K 2 (see page 224)
- Calm Sleep—B 62 (see page 218)
- High Mountains—B 60 (see page 219)

Diagrams of the location of these points can be found in Appendix A.

Yoga Facelift

In an advanced Yoga class, the facelift position involves standing on your head from thirty seconds to one minute. A novice would be required to kneel on the floor, forearms braced with the top of the crown of the head pressed against the floor. We are going to achieve the same results in a much less stressful way.

Benefits: This exercise increases circulation to the face and head. The result is a clearer mind, improved skin tone, and the reduction of fine lines and wrinkles.

Posture: Begin in the same position as in the previous exercises.

Visualization: Picture reversing the effect of the pull of gravity on your facial muscles. Imagine the increased flow of blood and energy to your brain.

Pathways: Energy will travel through the meridian that runs up the spine and the chongmei in the center of the body. The energy will return through the three dan tiens to the lower part of the abdomen.

1. Bend over from the hips so that your head is hanging down between your knees.
2. Allow your arms to dangle alongside your thighs.
3. Relax all the muscles of your face, lips slightly parted. You will be unable to breathe deeply during this time because your chest is resting on your thighs, so breathe lightly through your nose only.

4. Remain in this position for one minute if you are able to without becoming lightheaded or dizzy. If the position bothers you, reduce the time to thirty seconds and increase that time gradually as you become more comfortable in this position.

5. Regardless of the amount of time you spend in this position, breathe in as you return to your original posture by rolling yourself upward until your back is straight and against the back of the chair. Use your abdominal muscles to pull yourself upright.

Relax for a moment and check your posture before beginning the next exercise.

You may use any or all of the following points either before or after you do the Yoga Facelift exercise. These acupressure points are particularly effective if you have facial blemishes, eczema, hives or for bruises on any part of the body. To find their location, and for a description of the benefits provided by each healing point, turn to Chapter 5.

- **Facial Beauty**—St 3 (see pages 184, 205, 207, 213, 215)
- **Four Whites**—St 2 (see pages 205, 213)
- **Heavenly Pillar**—B 10 (see pages 188, 192, 205, 211, 228)
- **Sea of Vitality**—B 23 and B 47 (see pages 198, 213)
  Do not use these points if you have a fracture, broken bones in your back, or disintegrating discs. If you suspect that any of these conditions are present, see your physician before using these pressure points.
- **Three Mile Point**—St 36 (see pages 193, 197, 201, 213)
- **Third Eye Point**—GV 24.5 (see pages 187, 199, 205, 210, 228, 229)
- **Windscreen**—TW 17 (see pages 204, 214)

Diagrams of the location of these points can be found in Appendix A.

The following relaxation exercises can be done any time, anywhere, as long as you're in a fairly quiet environment. Once you become familiar with the technique, you may find yourself slipping into this peaceful frame of mind almost unconsciously. You can use this relaxation method at work to reduce stress, going into a quiet zone without leaving your desk. Used at bedtime, these exercises will help you fall quickly to sleep and ensure a restful, full night's sleep.

Wherever you have pain or discomfort, center your mind on that area and breathe into it. As you take a deep, diaphragmatic breath in through your nose, direct that cleansing oxygen to the part of your body that is giving you trouble. As you breathe out through your mouth, know that waste material is being expelled and, along with it, the blockage in the meridian or juncture point that was causing the soreness. As you concentrate on whole-body breathing, remember that the intake of oxygen is metabolizing unusable fat, destroying harmful bacteria, and revitalizing all your cells.

When you complete this relaxation section, treat yourself to an 8-ounce glass of water. Remember that it is very hard to tell when your body needs rehydrating. Setting a goal for yourself to drink so many ounces of water during your T'ai Chi session (based on how much water your are drinking the rest of the day) will help to ensure that you do not become dehydrated.

Return to your original posture, i.e., feet flat on the floor, legs approximately shoulder-width apart with your back flat against the chair. Take several deep breaths and feel yourself relaxing. Return to your mental image of a swift river. Reduce the waves on the surface of the water, gradually smoothing out the waves until the water is completely smooth and flowing without a ripple.

Now, close your eyes and concentrate on your head, facial muscles, and neck. Imagine the spot where the upper dan tien is located. Draw an imaginary line from the tops of your ears through the center of your skull. Then imagine another line running from the Third Eye Point straight to the back of your head. Where these two lines meet is the location of the upper dan tien. Take a deep breath in through your nose and expand your diaphragm pressing the ch'i into the lower abdominal area. Set it to spinning with your mind so that the velocity of that spin releases waves of energy upward to neck and head. Visualize the energy entering and circulating through this area as you take three deep breaths—in through your nose, out through your mouth, using your diaphragm to push the air in and out.

Move your attention downward, now, to your shoulders, arms and hands. Imagine the energy moving down from your neck and traversing the pathways, yangyumei, along the outside of your arms, through your hands and returning through the yinyumei on the inside of your arms and back to your shoulders.

Push the energy from your shoulders into the your trunk. Repeat the three deep, diaphragmatic breaths and direct the energy around and through the vital organs protected by your rib cage.

Breathe in through your nose and expand your diaphragm once again as you press the energy into your hips, down your thighs, and into the knee joint. The energy is passing along the yangqiaomei on the outside of the leg, circling the bottom of your kneecap and returning to the hip joints by way of the yinqiaomei on the inside of your leg.

Send the energy back down the outside of your leg, past the knee and into your calves, ankles and feet. Breathe into these areas, focusing particularly on any spot that is sore or where the muscles have become strained. The energy will then move naturally toward the ground, passing through and soothing the muscles and joints of your legs and feet.

Benefits: After you complete this section, your body will be relaxed, your mind clear, and your spirit restored to a state of balance and calm.

Posture: As in the previous exercises.

Visualization: Imagine yourself floating on a cloud as soothing energy passes from the top of your head, through your arms and trunk and, finally, into your legs from where it flows back into the earth.

Pathways: All the meridians of your body are addressed in this section creating an unobstructed flow of energy from head to toe.

1. Close your eyes. Take a deep breath and expand your diaphragm. Picture a flow of energy traveling up, down and through your head, neck and facial muscles.

Repetitions: Three calming breaths before focusing on the next part of your body.

2. With your mind, push the energy from your neck down into your shoulders, arms and hands while breathing deeply in and out, expanding and contracting your diaphragm.

   Repetitions: Three very deep, soothing breaths.

3. From your shoulders, press the stream of energy into your trunk. Allow the healing energy to circle in and around your organs and to travel up and down your spine.

   Repetitions: Three deep, healing breaths.

4. Now, push the energy from your trunk down into your hips, thighs and knees. Warm and soothe sore muscles and overworked joints by circulating the energy with your mind.

   Repetitions: Three deep, relaxing breaths.

5. Then, direct the energy that you have released with your thoughts and deep breathing into the lowest part of your legs, the calves, ankles, and, finally, the feet. Remember that we all exchange energy with our environment. Electromagnetic energy rises from the earth and is absorbed into the body through the soles of the feet. The energy coursing through our bodies is returned to the earth as it moves through our legs and out through the soles of our feet as well

   Repetitions: Three deep, energizing breaths.

ꙮ Centering Ch'i

Benefits: Centers the energy and rebalances the body.

Posture: As in the previous exercise.

Visualization: Imagine that you are collecting the ch'i and bits of energy from all over your body returning them to a neutral position at the lower dan tien so that none will be lost or trapped elsewhere in the body.

Pathways: You are targeting all the pathways you have used in the previous exercises.

1. Hold your hands palm up, just above your lap. Breathe in deeply through your nose while contracting your diaphragm. In this exercise, the diaphragm is **not** expanded during inhalations.

2. As you tighten your diaphragm and abdomen, raise your arms out to the side and up over your head to its center. Your palms are now facing the ceiling, fingers barely touching.

3. Allow your arms to descend gradually in an arc out to the side. As you do so, exhale until there is no breath left in your lungs and relax the muscles of your diaphragm and abdomen.

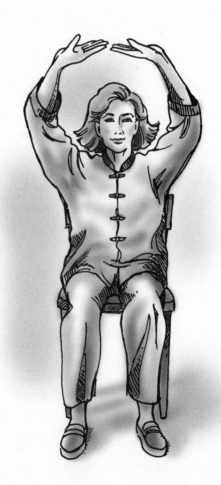

Centering Ch'i

4. Return your arms to the original position in front of the lowest part of your abdomen, palms facing upward.

Repetitions: Three

Stop and rest for a moment before getting up from your chair.

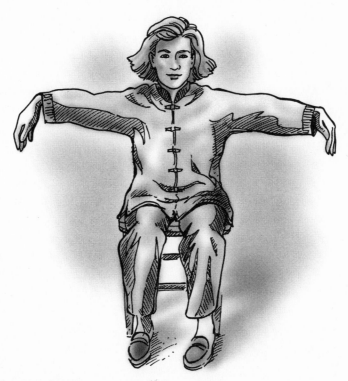

Centering Ch'i (continued)

Fifteen-Minute Daily Exercises: Introduction

If you are raising a family, pursuing a career, or devoting your time to aging parents, an hour set aside once or twice a week for T'ai Chi classes may be doable, but an hour a day for the complete set of exercises is not always possible. My friend, Mary Ann, found an ingenious way to make use of her knowledge of T'ai Chi. Stranded at an airport, her flight canceled, Mary Ann used T'ai Chi breathing, relaxation, and acupressure points to relieve her tension. A selection of upper- and lower-body exercises helped to reduce her anxiety and to alleviate the stiffness in her muscles and joints while she waited for hours for the airline to rebook her flight.

For busy people like Mary Ann, this chapter offers five fifteen-minute exercise programs that can be performed at work, at home, or even in an airport. When you practice these stretches at your desk during a break, you will return to your busy day calmed, centered, and refreshed. Put aside fifteen minutes in the morning to improve your performance throughout the day, or practice the stretches in the evening to ensure a restful night's sleep.

In this chapter, all the stretches from the full set of exercises are included but are broken up into fifteen-minute segments. Each of the segments includes the complete deep-breathing portion of the exercises and addresses either the internal organs or the upper- or lower-body muscles and joints. In addition, acupressure points are listed at the end of each set. Choose three of these points and use them before you go on to the next set. Each group of exercises concludes with part of the complete relaxation and mind centering exercises. To bring your body back into balance, Centering Ch'i always rounds off each of the sections.

Day one incorporates deep breathing with exercises for healing the internal organs. Massaging and squeezing the organs promotes the distribution of energy to these vital parts of the body. The twisting motions slim the waistline and trim the abdomen. Brushing Tree Trunk gives your midsection an excellent workout while balancing the right and left hemispheres of the brain.

Both the analytical and the intuitive portions of your brain are invigorated. The relaxation portion of day one covers massage and pressure points on the face and head. The Third Eye Point promotes creativity and, when used in conjunction with the pressure point GV 19, reduces sinus congestion and pain. The acupressure point GV 16 relieves nosebleeds, neck pain, and a sore throat.

Day two repeats the breathing section then moves on to the head, neck, and shoulders. Exercises are added to strengthen and stretch arms, trunk, hands, and waist. Reducing the waistline, toning the arms, and flattening the tummy are some of the benefits of these exercises. Peripheral vision is improved during the neck-loosening exercise while, in the relaxation portion of this chapter, arms and shoulders are massaged to improve circulation and reduce tension. In addition, acupressure points on the arms and hands stimulate the immune system, relieve frontal headaches, constipation, and depression. The pressure point LI 11 reduces the symptoms of a cold and the pain of arthritis in the elbow.

Upper-body exercises are continued on day three with Green Dragon and Plucking Thread to tighten and strengthen the muscles of the arms after the full complement of breathing exercises Following the movements of the hands and arms exercises the eye muscles. Trunk Rotation reduces the waistline while it limbers and strengthens the hip joints. In addition, abdominal muscles are tightened and the stomach flattened. The relaxation section stimulates the flow of energy from the top of your head to the bottom of your feet through concentration and deep breathing. This meditative sequence calms the spirit and clears the mind.

On day four, following the breath-control exercises, we begin addressing the needs of the muscles and joints of the lower body. Starting with Pushing Up Sky with Foot Rolls and ending with Loosening Knees, this set of exercises tones and defines the muscles of the lower leg and limbers the ankle joint and the foot while strengthening the surrounding muscles. Brushing the abdomen during the relaxation portion of this day's exercises regulates the bowels, reduces bloating, and trims the tummy area.

Massaging the hips and knees relieves the pain in those joints by increasing circulation and promoting the production of synovial fluid around the kneecap. Pressing and holding the acupressure point ST 36 reduces fatigue, benefits digestion, and stimulates the immune system. The pressure point Commanding Middle strengthens the lower back and knees while alleviating lower-back pain and sciatica.

After the body is fully oxygenated, day five continues with stretches for the lower body. All of the exercises trim and tone the thighs and flex and extend the hip and ankle joints. Sweeping Lotus promotes the production of lymphocytes to fight off viruses and the bacteria that cause infections. The Yoga Facelift helps to tone the complexion and bring color to the face by improving circulation while reducing fine lines and wrinkles. Day five ends, as did the exercises on day three, with a complete head-to-toe relaxation.

As you practice these stretches, feel free to substitute or add any acupressure points from Chapter 4 that target your particular needs. If you are adding several more pressure points, reduce the number of repetitions of one or more of the exercises to stay within the fifteen minute time frame. Increase the repetitions of any exercises that address an area of your body that you wish to strengthen or tone. However, because proper oxygenation is so important to overall health, it is recommended that you do the entire set of breathing exercises every day. Remember that as you work out and practice your deep breathing, toxins are being released.

These poisonous substances must be flushed from the body as soon as possible. Keep a large glass of water by your side and drink at least 8 ounces after each exercise session.

Fifteen-Minute Exercises: Day One

It is easy to hold what is still.
It is easy to plan for what has not begun.
Brittle things are easy to break.
Tiny things are easy to disperse.
Deal with things before they begin.
Establish order before disorder sets in.

—TAO TE CHING #64:1

Breathing Exercises

∾ Balloon Breathing

This exercise will cleanse the lungs and strengthen the muscle that is your diaphragm. You will be able to tell if you are breathing correctly by the in and out motion of your hands. Concentrate on the movement of breath as you relax gradually in time with your breathing. To further enhance your mood of calm, you may want to close your eyes. Take nine deep, expansive breaths. Visualize the ch'i or energy as it moves through your body. At the same time, and with the expansion of your diaphragm, remember to imagine ch'i as a spinning ball or disc. Bring the ball down into the lower part of your belly into the area known as the lower dan tien, which is approximately three finger widths below your belly button and about midway between your belly and your back. Think of yourself as purely skeletal without flesh or muscle. Imagine that there is a string attached to the top of your head holding you upward without any effort on your part. Begin to condense all the energy through the bones and into your marrow.

116

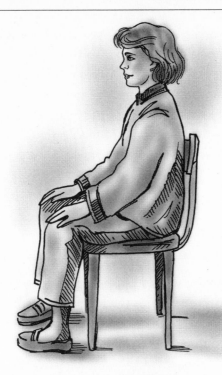

Posture

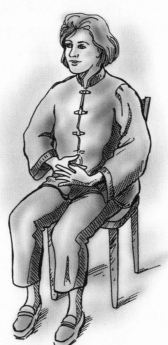

Balloon Breathing

117

❧ Flower Bud Opens

You will breathe in as you lift your arms over your head and arch your back. Concentrate again on the flow of energy to the marrow your bones while pressing the spinning ball downward. This exercise is like the big yawn-and-stretch movement you make when you first get out of bed in the morning. Your chest will be opened to its fullest extent clearing the stale air from your lungs and replacing it with clean, invigorating, fresh air. As your arms lower, exhale and stretch your arms out behind you as far as possible.

❧ Butterfly

During this exercise you are working to bring the energy into the center of your body and to center the ch'i into the lower dan tien. There is tension in the movement as you bring your arms forward together with your palms back to back. When you reach the full extension of the forward motion, swing your arms gently out to the sides in a full circle, reaching as far behind yourself as is comfortable. As you swing your arms out to the side, you will be completely relaxed while making your arms as weightless as you can. Remember that you are still suspended by the string attached to the top of your head and that you want the energy to flow through your bones and to their center.

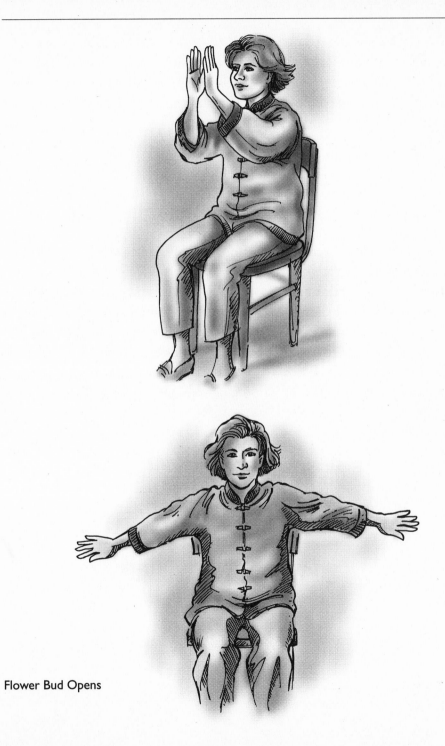

Flower Bud Opens

∾ Backward Arm Swings

This exercise will open your chest and allow your breath to move strongly into and out of your lungs. Be careful not to swing your arms too robustly since all T'ai Chi movements are supposed to be gentle and relaxed. Swing your arms back in sets of nine beginning with three or four sets, working up to a total of nine sets as soon as possible.

∾ Dragon's Breath

This is a wonderful exercise for warming the body and clearing the nasal passages. You should feel a significant burst of energy when you finish.

Breathe in slowly through your nose and exhale slowly also through your nose. Repeat three of these slow breaths. Then, inhale and exhale quickly eighteen times as though you were sneezing. After the eighteen "sneezes," pause for a second or two after each exhalation before inhaling again. Rest for a moment and then go on with another eighteen inhale/exhales. Slow your breathing down again by pausing between sets of inhale/exhale.

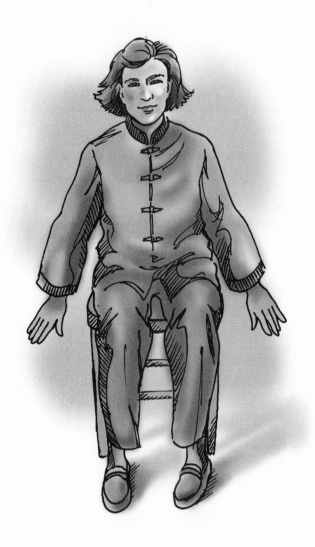

Backward Arm Swings

Acupressure Points for Improving Your Breathing

Choose three from this list:

Elegant Mansion

Use this point to relieve chest congestion, asthma, or coughing. It is **located** next to the breastbone in a hollow below the collarbone.

Fish Border

Use Fish Border to deepen breathing and relieve a swollen throat located in the middle of the thumb pad on the palm side of the hand.

Great Abyss

Use this point to clear the lungs, relieve coughing spasms, and the constriction of asthma. It is **located** below the base of the thumb in an indentation in the wrist.

Letting Go

Use this acupressure point to relieve breathing difficulties particularly when associated with emotional stress. It is **located** In the hollow below the collarbone and between the collarbone and the inside edge of the shoulder bone.

Lung Asscoiated Point

Use the Lung Associated Point to relieve sneezing and muscles spasms of the shoulders and neck which is **located** on your back, below the shoulder blade and between the spine and the scapula.

ꙮ Centering Ch'i

Check your posture again before beginning this final exercise, paying particular attention to toeing in with your feet and slightly rounding your shoulders. Hold your hands at a level three finger widths below your navel, palms upward, fingers almost touching. Circle your arms out to the side as you breathe in and tighten your diaphragm. This is known as *reverse breathing* and it is the exact opposite of the way you have inhaled in the previous exercises where you have deliberately and consciously expanded your diaphragm as you inhaled. This time, you are contracting diaphragmatic muscles as tightly as possible as you breathe in.

Raise your arms over your head so that both palms are facing the ceiling.

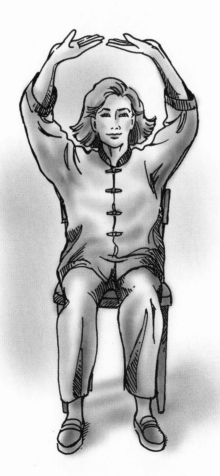

Centering Ch'i

Think of *condensing* your breath into the center of your body and pressing the spinning disc or ch'i into the lower dan tien as you inhale through your nose and raise your arms. Slowly exhale through your mouth and lower your arms in as relaxed a manner as you can without dropping them abruptly. Your hands should end with the palms up at the location of the dan tien, i.e., three finger widths below your belly button. Repeat the reverse breathing and arm raising with the palms turned toward the ceiling for a total of three times.

This exercise, as its name implies, is performed for the purpose of assuring that the ch'i or disc has been returned to its proper place, into the neutral

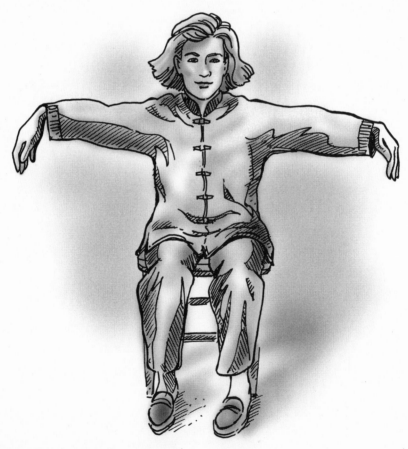

Centering Ch'i (continued)

zone. We do not want the ch'i to become trapped elsewhere in the body nor do we want it flowing in an uncontrolled way because that would throw the body out of balance.

By the time you have completed the first two or three exercises, you should begin to feel a tingling in your hands. With the proper amount of practice and concentration, that tingling will eventually spread out through your whole body. After a few months of consistent repetition of these exercises, you will begin to feel a sharper response to the centering of your ch'i. When you least expect it, you will feel as though you have received an electric shock. It may be localized on the tips of your fingers, somewhere on your leg or at the end of your toes. Remember that the *nonaction* of T'ai Chi is in the relaxed state of your muscles and joints. Bringing the ch'i into the lower dan tien and condensing the energy into the very marrow of your bones is a *mental* exercise.

If you feel yourself becoming tense while performing any of these exercises, stop and return either to the mental imaging of calming the water or to the opening exercise of deep, diaphragmatic breathing. Whichever you choose to do, remember the effort put forth in T'ai Chi is more mental than physical. There should be no excessive strain on the muscles in any of these movements but rather an application of thought and a steady concentration of the will on the targeted area.

Time: Approximately three minutes.

Healing Exercises

᭓ White Crane

As you perform this movement you are squeezing and massaging your kidneys, spleen, stomach, and liver. The four meridians that are located in your trunk are the pathways along which your energy will flow to these organs, nurturing and healing them. In addition, the twisting motion of the waist tightens and strengthens the abdominal muscles.

Breathe in through your nose, while you mentally press the ch'i into the lower dan tien as you swing your left arm down alongside your body with the palm facing the floor. Hold your right-hand palm facing forward alongside your right ear. Now, bring your right arm to the left, twisting your torso until the right hand is alongside the left ear while, at the same time, exhaling through your mouth. Twist to your right bringing your right hand down to your side with the palm facing the floor while your left hand reaches over to your right ear. Remember to breathe in through your nose as you begin the swing to the side and blow the air out through your mouth as you complete the twisting motion. Continue to alternate sides.

Repetitions: Eighteen

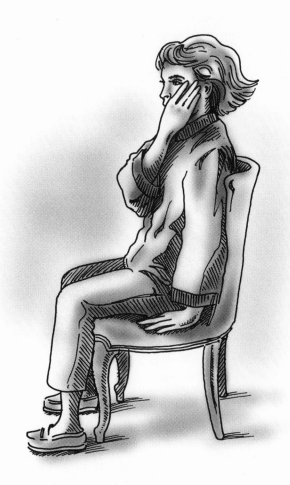

White Crane

~ Push Up Sky, Press Down on Earth

This exercise will stretch your arm muscles and lengthen and slim your waist-line. Think of the three meridians that travel up your spine, down the middle of your chest, and connect the lower *dan tien* with the middle of the top of your head. Concentrate on the energy flowing through them upward from the lower dan tien and downward from the upper dan tien.

Push your right arm up over your head with your palm facing the ceiling. At the same time, press your left arm down with the palm facing the floor. Breathe in through your nose and, as you do so, visualize the spinning disc that is the ch'i as sending out energy sparks throughout the upper and lower abdominal areas. Bring your arms together in front of your chest and exhale, tightening your chest and abdominal muscles and activating the power of the middle *dan tien*. Reverse and repeat again.

Repetitions: Eighteen

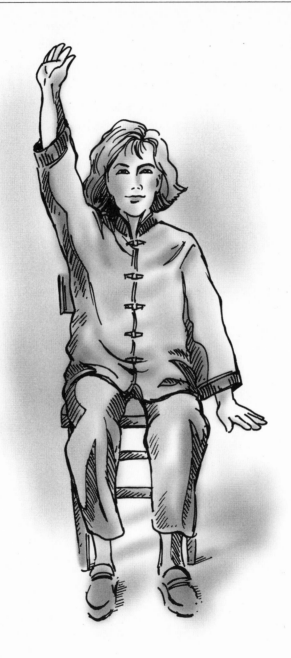

Push Up Sky/Press Down on Earth

∿ Turtle

This exercise is particularly beneficial for stretching the neck and shoulder muscles. In addition, this stretch strengthens the muscles of the abdomen and the diaphragm. The stronger your diaphragm, the deeper and more cleansing each breath will be. Tightening your abdomen will flatten your stomach.

Press both arms down by your sides, hands held flat with the palms toward the floor. Look up at the ceiling and breathe in through your nose, expanding your diaphragm to its fullest extent. Bring your hands to the middle of your chest. Think of yourself as a turtle pulling back into his shell as you bring your head down. Hunch your shoulders slightly and squeeze your stomach and chest muscles while exhaling.

Repetitions: Nine

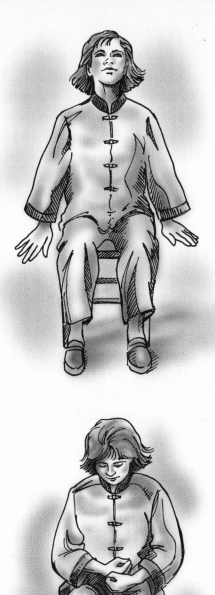

Turtle

In this exercise, you are targeting all three dan tiens through the connecting pathway known as the chongmei. With the swing of your arms from below the navel to the center top of your head, you are pulling the energy from the lower dan tien through the middle dan tien to the upper dan tien. In other words, with the movement of your arms up and down and the visualization of the energy moving in both directions through the centermost pathway, you are, in effect, forcing the energy to the top of your head and back down to the pubic bone.

Lace your fingers and swing your arms up over your head so that your palms are facing the ceiling. If this puts too much pressure on your arm and shoulder muscles, reverse your hands so that they are palm down. Breathe in as you raise your arms and blow out the breath as you lower your arms back to your lap.

On the ninth swing overhead, stop for a moment, lean to your right, overhead again and then lean to your left and so on, counting each lean as one. When you have completed nine leans, circle your arms in front of your upper chest, back up and down and around again for a total of nine times. Next, repeat the leans beginning to the left this time for the same number of repetitions and then circle again. Each time you move your arms overhead, bring them to the very center of your head where the upper dan tien is located. With your arms extended expand your diaphragm as much as possible and concentrate on the spinning ch'i disc in the lower dan tien. As you exhale and swing in an arc to the front, tighten your lower abdominal muscles forcing the energy to rise from the lower dan tien up through the solar plexus and on to the top of your head. Once again you will be stimulating and nurturing all your internal organs from the intestines through the upper chest.

Repeat the up-and-down movements, i.e., straight overhead and back down to your lap, for another total of nine swings. By this time your arms and shoulders may be feeling strained. If so, stop for a moment, take a couple of deep breaths and relax.

Repetitions: Nine

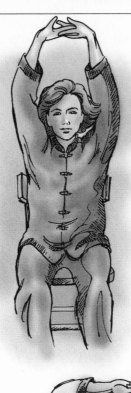

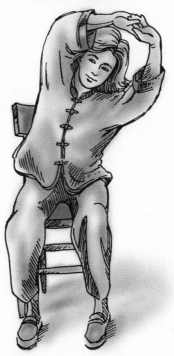

Holding Up Sky

133

∿ Brushing Tree Trunk

As you tighten your abdomen during this exercise, you will be releasing the energy into your chest and your arms. Looking in the opposite direction from the movement improves your coordination and your sense of balance. In addition, the movement of your head from side to side in opposition to the movement of your trunk equalizes the particular abilities of the right and left hemispheres of the brain.

Lift both arms as high as possible. Swing downward with one arm until it brushes the thigh on the opposite side. For example, if you swing to the left, your right arm will brush along your left thigh. At the same time look back over your right shoulder and upward.

All organs in the chest and abdomen are squeezed and massaged by the twisting motion of your waist. Additional energy is released along the outer pathway in your arms and back up the inner pathway to return the energy to your shoulders and down into your trunk. Take your time learning this exercise until you are confident that you are breathing correctly and that you are turning your head away from the direction in which you are twisting.

∿ An

Begin this exercise with your hands in front of your shoulders, palms facing outward. Twist to the left and push your hands out until your elbows are almost completely straight. Bring your hands back to their original position, twist to the right, and push out again. Continue alternately from side to side, breathing in when your hands are at your shoulders and breathing out as you push to the side for a total of eighteen times. Keep in mind that the Chinese word *an* refers to the type of pressure used by an experienced massage therapist. Use enough force to stretch your arm muscles, but don't overdo it.

Once again, it is vital that you expand your diaphragm to its fullest extent in order to release the energy from the spinning disc in the lower dan tien. The daimei is a significant pathway during this exercise as are the yangyumei and the yinyumei meridians, which are carrying the energy into and through your arms. After a few repetitions of this movement, you should be experiencing a fairly noticeable tingling in your hands. In addition, your waist is getting a considerable amount of action throughout this section. You should notice a change in its dimensions within a few weeks.

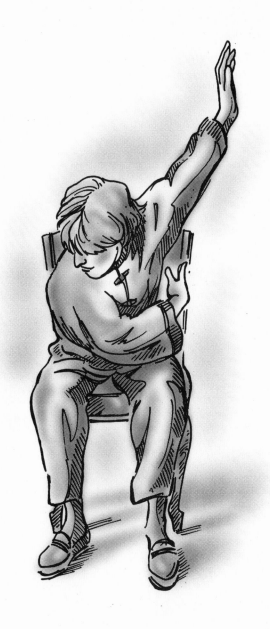

Brushing Tree Trunk

Acupressure Points for Healing

Choose any three of the following acupressure points:

Crooked Pond

Use this point to relieve constipation by stimulating the intestines and to strengthen your immune system. It is **located** at the outside edge of the elbow crease.

Heavenly Pillar

Use this point to reduce anxiety, stress, overexertion, and insomnia. It is **located** at a point $1/2$ inch below the base of the skull on the two large vertical muscles (trapezius).

Joining the Valley

Use this effective point to reduce the pain of a headache, to relieve constipation, and alleviate feelings of depression. This point is **located** between the thumb and index finger where the two fingers are joined.

Outer Gate

Use this acupressure point to reduce allergic reactions and relieve the pain of rheumatism and tendonitis. It is **located** between the two large arm bones (radius and ulna) two and a half finger widths away from the wrist crease toward the elbow.

Sea of Energy

Use this point to strengthen your lower back and to relieve gas and constipation. It is **located** two finger widths below your navel.

Sea of Tranquillity

Use this point to reduce feelings of nervousness, anxiety, depression, or hysteria. It is **located** on the breastbone three finger widths up from the base of that bone.

As you may remember, centering ch'i is a necessary conclusion to each section of exercises. We have moved the energy up and down through the chest and abdomen and out to the tips of the fingers and back again to the shoulders. It is important that we recenter this ch'i in case our spinning disc has become trapped somewhere in the body where it may stagnate or send too much energy to an area that we do not wish to target. Repeat three times before beginning the relaxation exercises.

Time: Approximately six minutes.

Relaxation Exercises

Rub your hands together to make them warm and palm your eyes. Cover your eyes at least three times and breathe naturally and deeply. Then, steeple your fingers at the Third Eye Point, which is located above the nose bone and between your eyebrows. Hold for thirty seconds. If your are experiencing sinus problems, hold your right hand at the crown of the head where you had a soft spot when your were a baby and a finger of your left hand at the Third Eye Point to relieve the pressure.

Next, gently pinch both your eyebrows sliding your fingers from the inside corner by your nose to the outside corner. Keep your eyes closed while you slide your fingers along your eyebrows nine times. Massage your temples upward and outward with your fingertips for a total of nine times. Then, place your hands on either side of your nose at the level of the nostrils and massage outward along your cheekbones to the outside edge of your eyes. Repeat again for a total of nine times. Now, place your fingertips on either side of your chin and move them in a circular motion upward and outward.

In Chinese medicine, the ear is thought to contain pressure points related to all the organs of the body. If you have a hearing aid, however, you will need to remove it or skip all of the following self-massage techniques involving the ears.

Though it may seem contradictory, rubbing your ears can be both stimulating and relaxing. Whenever you're sitting at your desk at work and begin to feel yourself nodding off, rub your ears briskly for a few seconds. You may be surprised to find yourself considerably energized. To further stimulate the important organs of the body, pull gently on your earlobes and then rub your thumbs up and down directly behind your ears. Next, press your palms against your ear and release, pressing again and releasing for a total of nine times.

With your mouth closed, circle your tongue nine times in one direction and then nine times in the other. Clench you front teeth together nine times and repeat with your back teeth on one side, then on the other side working your jaw muscles thoroughly. Be careful not to grind your teeth. The purpose of this exercise is to strengthen the jaw muscles and teeth.

Move your hands to the back of your head and find the area that the Chinese call the Wind Mansion. The Wind Mansion is a large depression located at the base of the skull. Press into this area with a moderate amount of pressure. Hold your finger on that point for thirty seconds. The Wind Mansion is beneficial for reducing the symptoms of a cold or the flu and for relieving depression. You will feel an almost immediate response from your sinuses as those cavities begin to loosen and drain.

Now, use the fingertips of both hands and tap your skull gently from the occipital area, along the center of your head all the way to the beginning of your hairline and then outward on each side in the general shape of the hemispheres of the brain. This tapping motion is thought to stimulate brain activity and if practiced regularly to prevent memory loss. Repeat down the center and around the sides for a total of nine times. Finish at the hairline and then press firmly on the eight bones of the skull beginning with the frontal bone.

The frontal lobe functions as the center for the higher order of brain activities such as planning, thinking, and worrying. This is also the impulse center and, if undamaged, regulates the ability to resist reckless behavior.

Press against the temporal bones above and behind the temples for about thirty seconds. The temporal lobe encased in the temporal bones are the center for speech and the processing of sounds. Damage to this area of the brain as the result of a stroke restricts the speech and comprehension ability of the stroke victim.

Next, locate the parietal bones, which are situated on each side of the upper part of the head between the frontal bone and the occipital bone moving laterally from front to back. The parietal lobe is responsible for conveying somatosensory information from the brain to the body, i.e., body awareness and kinesthesis, which is the perception of muscular movement.

Now, move your hands downward to the rounded bones behind your ears, the mastoids, and press against these bones with heels of your hands. If you have a sinus infection or a cold that affects your ears, this is a good place to press and rub to relieve the pressure and allow the ears to drain properly.

The occipital bone is the last of the series. You can find the occipital bone by placing your hands at the back of your head. The flattened area above the base of the skull is where you want to press. The occipital lobe controls vision.

If your arms are tired from holding them up to massage your face and head, take a moment to rest them before you start the next exercise. When you are ready, lace your fingers and place them at the back of your neck. Then, press your neck against your hands and release. The purpose of this exercise is to strengthen your neck muscles but has the added advantage of also working your arm muscles.

Repetitions: Nine presses and nine releases.

∽ Centering Ch'i

Repeat this exercise three times. Remember to use reverse breathing, to reach directly over your head and to lower your arms gently back to the lower dan tien.

Time: Approximately six minutes.

Fifteen-Minute Exercises: Day Two

A tree as big as an arm's breadth
begins as a small shoot.
A terrace nine tiers high,
begins as a handful of dirt.
An ascent to high places,
begins beneath one's feet.

—*Tao Te Ching, #64:2*

Breathing Exercises

Repeat all the breathing exercises from day one. Again, choose three acu-pressure points from the first day's section on breathing. Complete this section with three repetitions of Centering Ch'i.

Time: Approximately three minutes.

Upper-Body Exercises

∾ Head, Neck, and Shoulders

Visualize a person falling asleep while sitting in a chair. The sleeper's head bobs gradually downward until his chin is almost resting on his chest. This relaxed movement of the head is the feeling you should have as you tilt your head down. Lift your head back to the center (or upright on your spine) and then tip your head gently backwards, all in one fluid movement. Breathe in, using your diaphragm to pull the air in through your nose while your head is still in the upright position. As you lower your head, blow out through your mouth. The breathing pattern is the reverse when you lean your head back. Breathe in through your nose as your head tilts backward and then blow out through your mouth as you return your head to the upright position. Take in another breath and blow out as you bend your head toward your chest. Do nine sets of down, center, and back. Then, allow your head to tip to the side toward your shoulder. Center your head again, and then lean your head over the opposite shoulder for a total count of nine head tips to the shoulders. The breathing is the same here as it was with the downward motion. That is, take a breath in while your head is upright and let it out through your mouth as you lean to one side or the other.

On the ninth head tip, circle it down to your chest, to the opposite shoulder, then back to the upright position and repeat for nine half circles in the opposite direction. Bringing your ear toward your shoulder is again repeated for nine counts followed by nine half circles. Your breathing will not be as deep here as it was in the previous exercise. However, the same rule applies. Breathe in on the upright head position and out as you circle your head. At no time during the circling movement should you lean your head back: side to chest to side only.

When you have completed the neck stretches, lift your shoulders toward your ears, drop them, making them as limp as you can and then, lift them again. Shoulder shrugs should be performed slowly and to the fullest extent possible but without force. Count the entire up-and-down movement as one repetition and repeat for a total of nine times. Circle your shoulders back nine times and then forward nine times. Throughout the shrugs and shoulder circles, your arms and hands should dangle motionlessly and be completely relaxed.

∽ Wild Horse

Hold an imaginary basketball between your hands, palms facing one another with one hand directly over the other. Slowly raise the hand on the bottom upward and to the side while the other hand presses down and to the side. If, for example, your left hand is underneath and your right hand is on top. Slide your left hand up and to the left side until it is at eye level while, at the same time, moving your right hand with palm facing downward alongside your right thigh. Your eyes should follow your left hand (or whichever one is moving upward). Then, your left arm arches over your head as you lean to your right. The breathing follows the usual rule: breathe in when your arms are in front of your body and out as they move away from your chest. Breathe in again as your arm comes over your head and out, as you lean to the side. Think about the energy as it moves from the lower dan tien to the middle dan tien and up the spine into the arms. We are bringing energy from below the navel through the trunk and into the arms. When you have completed one set, reverse and repeat remembering to do this slowly and smoothly without strain or force.

Repetitions: Eighteen

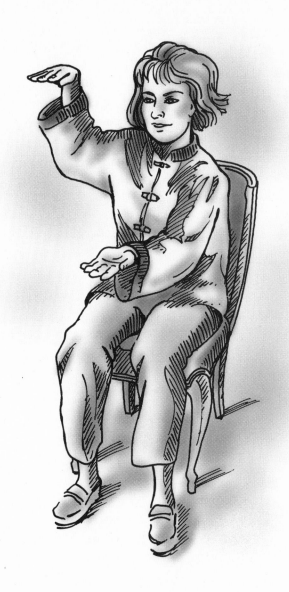

Wild Horse

∾ Bird's Feathered Hand

Bend your elbows and hold your hands fisted in front of your shoulders. Stretch one arm at a time out to the side, slowly open your fingers and feel the air as it passes through the spaces between your fingers. Close your hand gradually, compressing the molecules of air, and return your arm to its original position. Stretch out your other arm and repeat again for a total of eighteen times until you have completed an equal number on each side. During the entire exercise, think of the air through which your arms are moving, the molecules flowing in between your fingers and then, being squeezed out as you close your hand into a fist. Consider, too, how the energy is traversing shoulders and arms, down the outside of the arms through the hands, and returning to the shoulders.

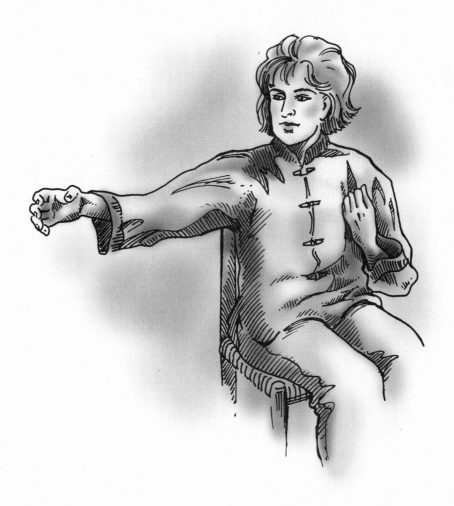

Bird's Feathered Hand

❧ Hands Waving in Clouds

This exercise benefits more than one area of the body. Your eyes are being exercised as they follow your upper hand from side to side. As you twist from side to side, your waist is being trimmed. In addition, the muscles of the upper arms, particularly in the area of the triceps, are tightening as you move your arms up and down, and back and forth.

This movement is performed just as its name implies. Think of yourself as parting a cluster of fluffy clouds in front of you. Both arms move in the same direction, one at eye level, the other at the level of the lower dan tien. The upper arm is held with the palm facing you while the lower arm is led by the inside of the wrist with the fingers trailing as you brush the imaginary clouds from in front of your face and abdomen. Your trunk should be moving with your hands, i.e., twisting to the side with the motion of your arms. Keep your eyes on the hand in front of your face so that your entire upper body is moving in unison.

Breathe in as you face forward and exhale as you twist to the side. The direction of the movement is determined by the upper hand so that if your left hand is level with your eyes, the movement will be to the left, and so on. Again, this movement should be repeated for a total of eighteen counts in order to provide an equal number on each side.

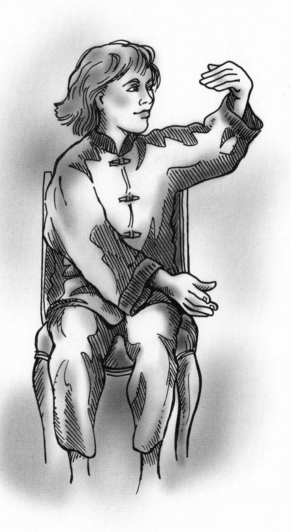

Hands Waving in Clouds

Acupressure Points for the Upper Body

Choose any three of the following:

Above Tears

Use this potent point to reduce hip pain, tension in the shoulder, and water retention. It is **located** in the space between the bones of the fourth and fifth toes on top of the foot.

Big Mound

Use this effective point to reduce the discomfort of carpal tunnel syndrome, rheumatism, and tendonitis in the wrist. It is **located** in the middle of the wrist crease on the inside of the arm.

Bigger Stream

Use this point for the pain of an infected wisdom tooth, for earaches, and ringing in the ears. It is **located** at the halfway mark between your inside anklebone and your Achilles' tendon.

Ear Gate, Listening Place, and Reunion of Hearing

Use this acupressure point for relief of toothaches, headaches, and pressure inside the ear. These three points are **located** in front of the ear with the Listening Place directly in front of the ear opening and the other two points ½ inch above and below the Listening Place.

Facial Beauty

Use this point to reduce eye fatigue or eyestrain as well as nasal and head congestion. It is **located** on the cheekbones directly below the pupils of the eyes.

Windscreen

Use this point to effectively reduce ear or jaw pain, a swollen throat, or toothaches. It is **located** in a small hollow behind the earlobe.

∽ Centering Ch'i

Refer to day one exercises for a description of this centering exercise. Repeat Centering Ch'i three times slowly.

Repetitions: Three

Time: Approximately five minutes.

Relaxation Exercises

∽ Thymus

The Chinese refer to this gland as the youth gland and consider its stimulation essential to fight off illness and retain youthful vitality. Press or circle your finger clockwise at the small indentation directly below the V of your collarbone for at least thirty seconds.

∽ Shoulders and Arms

With your opposite hand, brush your fingers from the back of your shoulder and down past your shoulder blade in the way that warm water flows over your shoulder when you are taking a shower. Still on the same side, run your hand down the outside of your arm from your shoulder, over your hand through the middle finger, pausing for a moment at the laogong junction point. The laogong point is located where the middle finger touches the palm when fisting your hand. Slide your working hand up the inside of the arm along the yinyumei meridian back to the shoulder. Repeat the running water and the arm strokes for a total of nine times for each, and then change sides.

Find the Shoulder Well point by measuring three finger widths from the base of the neck on the very top of the shoulder where the large muscle is located. Not only does this pressure point relieve insomnia but it is also beneficial for poor circulation, particularly in the hands and feet. If you have been diagnosed with chronic fatigue syndrome, this point may help to reduce the symptoms of that disease. Of course, it is not meant to replace medications or any other treatments recommended by your doctor.

Next, fold your arms and press a fingertip on the top of your arm at the end of the elbow crease (see page 185). Hold for approximately thirty seconds. This point is called the Crooked Pond and is beneficial for relieving constipation by stimulating the intestines.

On the inside of your wrist at the end of the crease directly below the little finger is a pressure point called Spirit Gate. This point relieves cold sweats and general anxiety as well as insomnia resulting from overexcitement. Use this point when you are having difficulty falling asleep after a stressful day or the night before your big interview.

Now, firmly press the flap of skin between your index finger and your thumb reaching to just in front of the area where the bones of the finger and thumb meet (see page 185). Hold for thirty seconds, then change hands and repeat. Use this pressure point if you are experiencing a frontal headache.

Wash your hands using the same motion as you do when you are actually using soap and water until they feel warm and relaxed. A word of caution: if you have a joint that is sore and arthritic, treat it gently. Do not pull on it or press too hard. With the opposite hand, press upward on each finger bringing the blood to the tip. Change hands and repeat. Take hold of each finger with your opposite hand and circle it gently to loosen the large knuckle joint. Once again, change hands and repeat. Now, play an imaginary piano, making certain that you separate each finger as you press down on the keys.

∾ Centering Ch'i

Refer to day-one exercises for a description of this exercise. Repeat three times slowly and thoughtfully.

Repetitions: Three

Time: Approximately seven minutes.

Fifteen-Minute Exercises: Day Three

At birth, a man is weak and flexible.
At death, he is hard and rigid.
All living things such as grass and trees,
are supple and yielding while alive,
and withered and dry when they die.
Thus, unyielding rigidity is the companion of death,
and yielding flexibility is the companion of life.

—*Tao Te Ching #76:1*

Breathing Exercises

Refer to day-one breathing exercises. Choose three acupressure points from the list on day one after you complete the last breathing exercise. Don't forget to do three repetitions of Centering Ch'i at the end of this section before beginning the upper-body exercises.

Time: Approximately three minutes.

Upper-Body Exercises

∿ Green Dragon

Bring your hands closer together over your right shoulder so that your left hand cups your right shoulder and your right hand is level with your right ear. Move both arms over your shoulder as though you are holding a bag (a very light one, remember) and then, swing it toward the floor. When you finish the movement, however, your right hand will remain at lower chest level while your left pushes down toward the floor to the side of your left thigh. Your right hand is held in a position that is called a knife hand in the martial arts, i.e., perpendicular to your body so that the hand is turned edgewise. At this point, tense the muscles in both arms. Prior to this final position, your arm muscles should have been loose and relaxed. Now, move your arms left so that your left hand is level with your ear and your right is close to your left shoulder. Repeat the swing of your arms slowly and with fluidity, alternating sides until you complete a total of eighteen Green Dragons.

Inhale through your nose as your arms come over your shoulder, and exhale through your mouth when your hands come to rest in the knife-hand position.

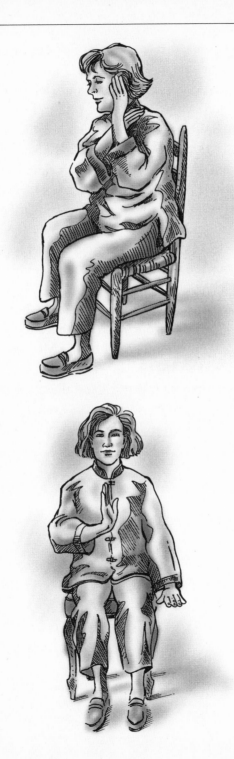

Green Dragon

～ **Repulse Monkey**

If you have completed the correct number of repetitions in the previous exercise, your left hand will be in the knife-hand position. Turn your hand so that the palm is facing up while swinging your right arm over and close to your right shoulder. Follow the direction of your right arm with your eyes by turning your head to look over your shoulder. Breathe in through your nose as your arm swings back and your head turns. Exhale through your mouth as you bring your right arm forward. Slide your right hand over your left so that the palms are about 1 inch apart, and press forward with your right hand pulling your left arm back and toward your side. Then, swing your left hand over your left shoulder as you turn your right hand palm up, and repeat the slide of one hand over the other with palms facing. Repeat this exercise for eighteen counts or at least for an equal number of repetitions with each hand.

Concentrate on pushing the energy through the outside pathway of the arm into the laogong point on your palm and back to the shoulder through the inside arm meridian. If you practice Repulse Monkey slowly enough and with sufficient attention to the movement of the energy through the two meridians and the juncture point, you will feel the exchange of heat from one hand to the other. As you progress with these exercises, you will eventually feel a startling amount of friction between your two hands.

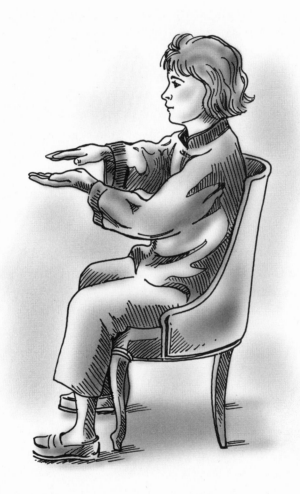

Repulse Monkey

❧ Plucking Thread

This exercise provides a tremendous pull of energy to your intuitive center. Plucking Thread is also an effective exercise for strengthening and sculpting the upper arms.

Begin this exercise with your hands on your thighs. One hand reaches down between your knees, then pulls an imaginary thread up to slightly above eye level. The same hand reaches down again to pull up another thread, and so on until you have pulled nine threads. As you do so, imagine the energy moving down the yangyumei meridian on the back side of your arm, moving through your middle finger and laogong junction on your palm back up through the inside pathway of your arm, the yinyumei. In your mind, draw the energy from the huiyin junction between the legs to and through the lower dan tien to the middle dan tien, stopping at the upper dan tien which is just above eye level. Consider the amount of energy being discharged from the major meridian juncture, the huiyin. All that power being generated by the spinning ch'i in the lower dan tien, rises to the intuitive, creative, and spiritual Third Eye Point.

Now, change arms and repeat on the other side. Finally, both arms reach down together and rise to the Third Eye Point together for a total of nine two-handed movements.

❧ Trunk Rotation

In this exercise you will be loosening and relaxing your hip joints. With the very deep breaths that accompany the trunk rotations, you will have made it possible for the lymphatic system to filter out excess fats and proteins and to rid your body of waste matter. The circular movement will trim your waistline.

Take a deep breath and expand your diaphragm and abdomen. Then lean to one side and circle your trunk so that your chest brushes your thighs. Breathe out as you lower your trunk and begin to breathe in again as you return to the upright position. Repeat for nine circling movements to the right and nine to the left.

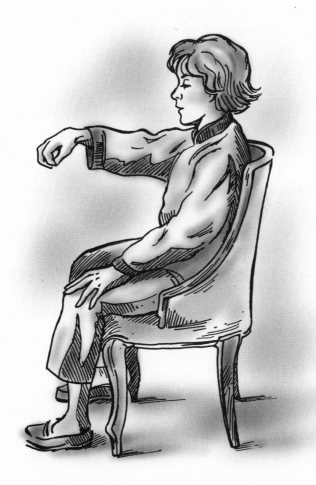

Plucking Thread

More Acupressure Points for the Upper Body

Choose any three of the following:

Bigger Rushing

Use this acupressure point to reduce the effects of allergies, headaches, and eye fatigue. It is **located** in the depression between the big toe and the second toe on the top of the foot.

Drilling Bamboo

Use this effective point to reduce red and painful eyes as well as clouded vision and hay fever. To **locate** this point find the indentations at the inner edge of the eyebrows on either side of the bridge of the nose.

Four Whites

Use this point to reduce facial blemishes. It is **located** in an indentation one finger width below the cheekbone in line with the iris of the eye.

Gates of Consciousness

Use this point to reduce stiffness of the neck, for dizziness, eyestrain, or irritability. To **locate** this point, run your finger along the base of your neck until you find a hollow between the two sets of vertical neck muscles (trapezius and sternoclineidomastoids).

Heavenly Appearance

Use this potent point to improve the tone of the skin and to relieve the itching and swelling of hives. It is **located** behind the jawbone in a hollow below the earlobe.

Wind Mansion

Use this acupressure point to reduce sinus and nasal congestion as well as for a sore throat or a headache. It is **located** in a large hollow at the base of the skull at the top of the spinal column (basal ganglia).

∾ Centering Ch'i

Refer to day one to refresh your memory about the reverse breathing and arm movements for this exercise.

Repetitions: Three

Time: Approximately five minutes.

Relaxation Exercises

∾ Head-to-Toe Relaxation

The following relaxation exercises can be done anytime, anywhere, as long as you're in a fairly quiet environment. Once your become familiar with the technique, you may find yourself slipping into this peaceful frame of mind almost unconsciously. You can use this relaxation method at work to reduce stress, going into a quiet zone without leaving your desk. Used at bedtime, these exercises will help you fall quickly to sleep and ensure a restful, full night's sleep.

Return to your original posture, i.e., feet flat on the floor, legs approximately shoulder-width apart with your back flat against the chair. Take several deep breaths and feel yourself relaxing. Return to your mental image of a swift river. Reduce the waves on the surface of the water, gradually smoothing out the waves until the water is completely smooth and flowing without a ripple.

Now, close your eyes and concentrate on your head, facial muscles, and neck. Imagine the spot where the upper dan tien is located. Draw an imaginary line from the tops of your ears through the center of your skull. Then imagine another line running from the Third Eye Point straight to the back of your head. Where these two lines meet is the location of the upper dan tien.

Take a deep breath in through your nose and expand your diaphragm pressing the ch'i into the lower abdominal area. Set it to spinning with your mind so that the velocity of that spin releases waves of energy upward to neck and head. Visualize the energy entering and circulating through this area as you take three deep breaths—in through your nose, out through your mouth using your diaphragm to push the air in and out.

Move your attention downward, now to your shoulder, arms, and hands. Imagine the energy moving down from your neck and traversing the pathways along the outside of your arms, through your hands and returning through the pathways on the inside of your arms and back to your shoulders. Push the energy from your shoulders into your trunk. Repeat the three deep, diaphragmatic breaths and direct the energy around and through the vital organs protected by your rib cage.

Breathe in through your nose and expand your diaphragm once again as you press the energy into your hips, down your thighs and into the knee joint. The energy is passing along the pathway on the outside of the leg, circling the bottom of your kneecap and returning to the hip joints by of the pathway on the inside of your leg.

Send the energy back down the outside of your leg, past the knee, and into your calves, ankles, and feet. Breathe into these areas, focusing particularly on any spot that is sore or where the muscles have become strained. The energy will then move naturally toward the ground passing through and soothing the muscles and joints of your legs and feet.

With your eyes still closed, mentally place yourself in a hot-air balloon of any color, size, and shape your desire. There you are, safely tucked in the basket with the colorful envelope holding you aloft as you sail through the clear blue sky with only the birds for company. As you float far above the earth, breathe in and out through your nose only, expanding and contracting your diaphragm. Relax and rest.

ꙮ Centering Ch'i

As usual, we end this day's exercise program with a final centering exercise. If you need to refresh your memory, consult day one. Remain seated for a minute or two after performing three centering movements.

Fifteen-Minute Exercises: Day Four

Constancy yields insight.
Lack of constancy yields disaster.
Insight leads to enlightenment,
enlightenment leads to impartiality,
impartiality leads to power,
power leads to oneness with nature,
oneness with nature leads to the Tao.
When eternally with the Tao,
one will not come to harm throughout life.

—*Tao Te Ching #16:2*

Breathing Exercises

Refer to day-one breathing exercises for a description and repeat them all before you begin the lower-body exercises. Choose three of the acupressure points listed after the breathing exercises for day one. Complete this section of exercises with Centering Ch'i.
Time: Approximately three minutes.

Lower-Body Exercises

∾ Pushing Up Sky with Foot Rolls

Lift your hands from your thighs, raising them overhead, palms toward the ceiling while, at the same time, pressing up on to the balls of your feet. Take a deep breath and expand your diaphragm. Visualize the spinning disc at the lower dan tien sending out waves of energy. These waves pass through your abdomen, trunk, and arms. At the same time, energy is traveling from the lowest juncture between the legs and halfway between the genitals and the anus through the outer pathway of your legs to your feet.

Bring your arms down to your sides, palms facing the floor and rock back on to your heels. Think of this movement as pulling your toes toward your ankles. Imagine the energy as it rises from the soles of your feet, up the inside of your leg through the huiyin, and back to the lower dan tien. Repeat for nine sets of ball to heel, arms pushing overhead and pressing down.

Repetitions: Nine

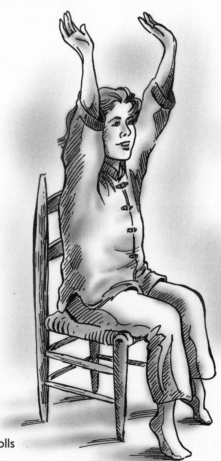

Pushing Up Sky with Foot Rolls

◠ Ankle Presses and Circles

Roll your feet back and forth from the balls to the heels nine times. Lift your feet off the floor, alternately pointing and flexing your feet nine times. With your feet still off the floor, circle each foot nine times in an inward direction. Change feet and repeat for the same number of times with the opposite foot. Return to the first foot and reverse the direction of the circle. Then, repeat again with the other foot.

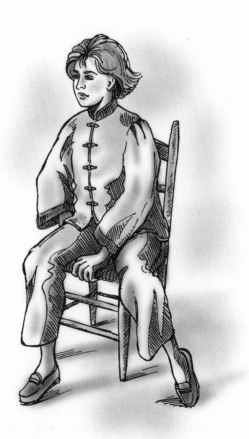

Ankle Circles

Place your feet back on the floor and press one foot at a time on to the ball, hold for a slow count of nine, then roll back on to the heel for the same amount of time. Lean slightly forward from the trunk to place more pressure on the ankle and the foot. Remember, this is a resistance exercise. Change feet and repeat.

Now, slide your leg out to the side of your chair, resting the foot on your big toe and relax your ankle completely. Circle your heel nine times in one direction and then nine times in the other. Change legs and repeat the heel circling for an equal number of times first in one direction then in the other.

Lift both feet off the floor and shake out your feet, holding them loose and relaxed. Treat your feet as though they were only loosely connected to the ankle. If you think too hard about shaking your feet, you'll defeat the purpose. This is a relaxing exercise intended to relieve any residual tension in the muscles of the lower leg.

∾ Loosening Knees

Sit slightly forward on your chair, with your hands on your knees, feet, and knees together. Circle your knees first in one direction then in the other (nine times each way). This may appear difficult at first because you are sitting down rather than standing. The trick here is to completely relax your legs from the hips down. Your ankles will also need to be as loose as possible. Since we just relaxed the ankles in the previous exercise, those joints should move easily. Your hands will provide additional help to guide your knees in a circular motion. Try not to move your upper body any more than is absolutely necessary. The emphasis should be entirely on the movement of the knees.

When you have completed nine circles in each direction, use your hands to push your knees gently, but firmly, apart. Allow them to close together again and repeat for nine pushes and returns. Your feet must remain flat on the floor, however, while you are pushing your knees out to the side so you will not get the maximum inner thigh stretch. Think of this knee push as priming the pump for the Chair Straddles that follow on day five.

Acupressure Points for the Lower Body

Choose any three from the following acupressure points. Press and hold on each point for thirty seconds.

Commanding Middle

Use this potent point to strengthen the lower back and to relieve stiffness and pain in your knees. It is **located** in the middle of the crease at the back of your knee.

Grandfather Grandson

Use this point to stop diarrhea, relieve indigestion, a stomachache, or nausea. It is **located** one thumb width behind the ball of the foot on the arch of the foot.

High Mountains

Use this acupressure point to reduce swollen feet, lower-back pain, and relieve pain in ankles or thighs. This point is **located** on the outside of the ankle in the hollow midway between the ankle bone and the Achilles' tendon.

Middle of a Person

Use this point for first aid in dealing with dizziness, fainting, and cramps. It is **located** directly below the base of the nose bone.

Supporting Mountain

Use this potent point to relieve cramps in the calf of the leg, for swollen feet, and knee pain.

Travel Between

Use this acupressure point for a headache or diarrhea. It is **located** at the joint between the big toe and the second toe.
Time: Approximately nine minutes.

Relaxation Exercises

ᨄ Abdomen, Hips, and Lower Back

The purpose in this abdominal exercise is to move the energy downward from the upper body and back to the lower dan tien. The warmth of your hands will be soothing for the abdominal muscles as well and is helpful for bloating and constipation.

Beginning in the region of your stomach and using both hands one on top of the other, press firmly as you slide your hands over your abdomen. Continue to press and slide over stomach and abdomen for a total of twenty-seven times (or three sets of nine).

The hip is a ball-and-socket joint. The ball of the joint is actually the spherical head of the femur. By massaging this area, we are not only bringing a soothing touch to the hip itself but also promoting the movement of energy down and through the leg. Aging is often the cause of pain and stiffness in the hip joints as the coating of cartilage and the flow of synovial fluid is reduced. Massaging the hip on a daily basis can relieve these symptoms. With both hands moving in a circular motion back to front, massage each hip twenty-seven times (see page 102). The pressure should be firm but not too hard. If you have consistent pain or stiffness in your hip, experiment with the number of rubs and the frequency of the massage sessions to see which appears to be most helpful for your particular condition. Of course, always consult your primary-care physician if you have an injury or if there is any possibility that the joint has deteriorated.

One of the most common complaints heard today is that of lower-back pain. It is an easy area to reach and you should be able to massage your lower back effectively. Run your fingertips up and down your back at least nine times. If your back is particularly painful you may need to use the palm and heel of your hands to relieve the soreness.

Beginning at the top of your thigh and using fingertip pressure, run one hand along the outside of your leg. Slide your hand over the top of your foot and middle toe and down to the yongquan point on the sole of your foot between the middle toe and the heel behind the ball of the foot. With your other hand, run your fingers firmly up the inside of your leg tracing the path of the yinqiaomei meridian to the upper thigh. Massage your leg nine times, and then repeat on the other leg.

The knee joint, like the hip joint, is prone to injury and overuse as well as the degenerative processes of aging. The hingelike motion of the knee depends on healthy cartilage and on the amount of synovial fluid that exists in the joint. Physical activity is essential to maintaining the health of the knees. Small injuries and wear and tear, however, are common and massaging this important joint will keep it more pain free and flexible.

Circle each kneecap from the outside to the inside using both hands. Change knees and repeat for a total of thirty seconds on each knee. Make sure that your hands are warm and that you exert a firm, but not excessive, pressure. The circular motion of your hands may stimulate the production of synovial fluid and will certainly relax and soothe the muscles and ligaments that surround the knee.

Now, lay your fingers on the outside bottom edge of your knee and measure three finger widths down. This is the Three Mile acupressure point for relieving nausea and fatigue. You should feel a good sized depression in this area (see page 193). Press a fingertip firmly on the top of this depression at the curved arch of the bone. You may press on both legs at the same time for at least thirty seconds.

At the back of the knee in the middle of the crease is an acupressure point called the Commanding Middle. Press on this point with your thumbs for a minimum of thirty seconds. Lean forward from the waist to give yourself more leverage. By using this pressure point, we are also furthering the flexibility of the knee joint itself.

❧ Yoga Facelift

Sit in your usual beginning position, feet flat on the floor shoulder-width apart, back against the back of your chair. Lean over so that your head is between your knees, arms dangling on either side of your legs. Your chest and abdomen will be resting on your thighs. Relax all the muscles of your face, lips slightly parted. Breathe through your nose. Remain in this position for thirty seconds for the first few practices. After that, gradually increase the time to a one minute. You may reduce the amount of time if you become dizzy in this position or have difficulty breathing. Unless you have a serious condition, the symptoms will go away as you repeat this exercise over a period of time. Regardless of the amount of time spent with your head hanging down, breathe in as you return to a sitting position and come up *slowly*. Take a moment to reorient yourself, and then begin the final centering exercise.

❧ Centering Ch'i

Remember to use reverse breathing for this exercise. Pull in on your abdomen and tighten your diaphragm when you take a deep breath. Always lower your arms more slowly than you raised them.

Repetitions: At least three.

Time: Approximately three minutes.

Fifteen-Minute
Exercises: Day Five

Attain the utmost emptiness.
Maintain the deepest stillness.
All things rise to activity,
and I watch their return.
They come forth and flourish,
then return to their origin.
Returning to one's origin is stillness.
Stillness is the fulfillment of one's nature.
Fulfilling one's nature is to be constant.

—TAO TE CHING #16:1

Breathing Exercises

Repeat all of the day-one breathing exercises. Once again, choose three acupressure points from the list that follows the breathing section for the first day. Press and hold on each of your chosen acupressure points for thirty seconds. End this portion of today's exercises with Centering Ch'i.
Time: Approximately three minutes.

Lower-Body Exercises

∾ Chair Straddles

This exercise will stretch the muscles on the inside of the thighs while contracting the muscles on the outside. The result is slimmer, firmer thighs.

Before you begin this exercise, return to your original position with your back pressed against the back of your chair, hips tucked under, and legs shoulder-width apart. Straddle your chair by first moving one leg out to the side and then the other. Hold for a couple seconds, and then return your legs to the front of the chair. Be careful not to arch your back or slump as you stretch the inside of your thighs. This is exactly like a leg stretch on the floor except that your knees are bent rather than straight. The feeling of truly stretching those muscles is important. However, do not overstrain. To prevent injury and loosen what may be overly tight muscles, breathe into the straddle. Inhale deeply while your legs are still in front of the chair. As you begin to move the first leg out to the side, slowing blow out your breath so that you are still exhaling when the second leg reaches the side and during the short hold time. This will allow you to move your legs further back without strain. Return to your original position, legs in front of the chair, shoulder-width apart in preparation for the next exercise.

⌒ Bow Stance

In this exercise, we are once again trimming and toning the leg muscles from the thigh through the calves and into the ankle.

Turn yourself so that you are seated diagonally on your chair, legs close together. Stretch your outside leg behind you and straighten your knee. Let's say, for example, that you turned yourself diagonally left. Then it will be the right leg that will be extended to the back. In addition to straightening your knee, your foot must remain flat on the floor. This will require your ankle to be bent over the inside of your foot elongating the muscles, tendons, and ligaments on the outside of your leg. To ensure that your foot stays flat on the floor, try sliding your foot out to the side and back. If you can't quite straighten your knee at first, don't worry. With practice, you will be able to do so.

Learning how to breathe into the movement will be helpful for a maximum stretch. Inhale while both legs are together at the corner of the chair. Begin exhaling slowly as you slide your leg back. Inhale as you return the leg to its original position. Then, turn diagonally right and repeat with the left leg stretched out behind you. Remember to inhale as you turn to the opposite corner of the chair and exhale slowly as you extend the left leg. Try not to roll over onto the inside of that foot.

Repetitions: Eighteen, alternating legs each time.

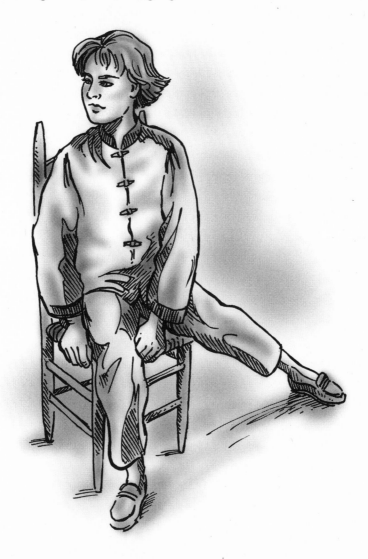

Bow Stance

Keeping your back pressed against the chair, lift one leg, knee bent and toe pointed downward. Hold the leg up for a slow count to six. Breathe in as you lift your leg, expanding your diaphragm. Consider the direction of the energy flow. By inhaling deeply you will be pressing the ch'i once again into the lower dan tien, which, in turn, will stimulate the distribution of energy through the working leg. Exhale as you lower your leg and tighten your abdominal muscles, lifting up on your rib cage. Hold for a slow count to six. Then, release, breathing in and inflating your diaphragm as you lift the other leg as you are able. Hold for a slow count of six, then lower your leg, exhaling again. Tighten your abdominal muscles again and hold for another six counts. Repeat the leg lifts nine times on each side for a total of eighteen lifts.

If you have one leg that is stronger than the other, which is not at all unusual, don't lift it much higher than the weaker one. Remember, throughout all of these exercises, we are not only trying to enhance the flow of energy throughout our bodies but we are also attempting to balance the yin and yang. An uneven number of repetitions on one side or the other, a greater stretch, or a higher lift constitute an imbalance in the exercise. You must work out a compromise between the strong leg (or arm or shoulder) in order to benefit both. Ask more of the weak side and a little less of the stronger side. Otherwise, there is the real possibility that you will overstrain muscles or gain greater strength on the stronger side while losing it on the weaker side.

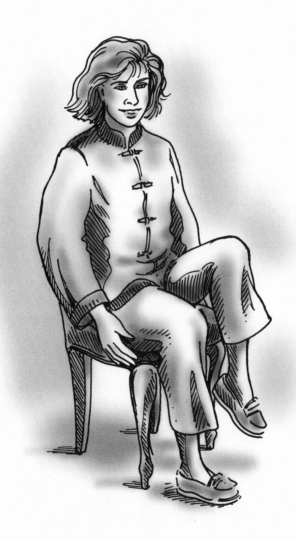

Golden Cockerel Stands on One Leg

Reaching for the Needle at the Bottom of the Sea is a metaphor for delving into the subconscious in the search for creativity. The early Taoists might not have expressed the metaphor in these exact terms but they surely realized the difficulty involved in any creative effort. As you practice this movement, visualize lifting that intuitive, creative power from the bottom of the sea as you reach for the floor and then returning with it to the upright position.

Like the preceding exercise, this one takes some getting used to if you have not been exercising on a regular basis. Begin in the standard posture—back against the chair, hips tucked slightly under you. Stretch one leg out to the front with a straight knee.

Using the opposite hand, stretch down to the floor between your legs. Breathe in as you lift your leg and exhale as you reach toward the floor. This breathing pattern will allow you to reach farther with less strain on your back.

Repetitions: Nine with each leg for a total of eighteen.

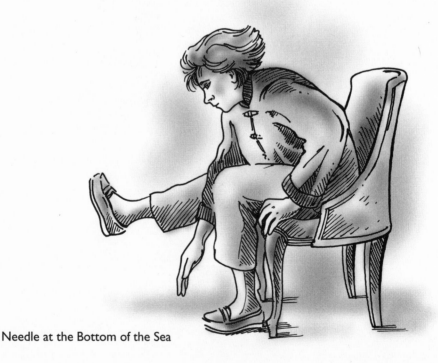

Needle at the Bottom of the Sea

∽ Leg Sweeps Lotus

Leg Sweeps Lotus is situated immediately after Needle at the Bottom of the Sea for a very good reason. It is a relaxed exercise and is intended to rid your legs, hips, and back of any discomfort caused by the previous exercise. Leg Sweeps Lotus not only works the muscles of your legs but also loosens the hip joints. In addition, the cross-over movement stimulates the lymph nodes that are in the groin area.

As the name implies, one leg sweeps over the other. Because we are seated, the working leg will brush lightly over the thigh of the unmoving leg. The knee of the working leg should be kept as straight as possible. Reverse and repeat.

Repetitions: Nine with each leg for a total of eighteen.

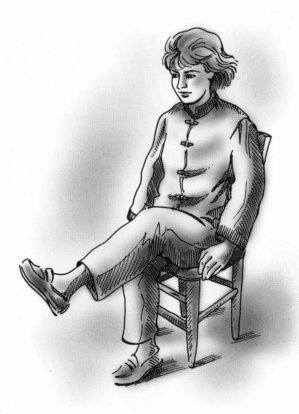

Leg Sweeps Lotus

More Acupressure Points for the Lower Body

Choose any three of the following:

Blazing Valley

Use this acupressure point to reduce swelling, particularly in the feet. It is **located** on the inside of the foot at the highest point of the arch midway between the big toe and the back of the heel.

Calf's Nose

Use this potent point to reduce pain, stiffness, or swelling of the knee. It is **located** on the outside of the leg in a hollow directly below the kneecap.

Sea of Vitality

Use this point to relieve lower-back aches and sciatica. It is **located** at two points on either side of the spine. The first point is two finger widths from the spine while the second point is four finger widths away from the spine. These two points are in line with each other between the second and third lumbar vertebrae.

Shady Side of the Mountain

Use this point to alleviate leg cramps and the pain of varicose veins. It is **located** below the knee on the inside of the leg directly under the large bulge of the bone.

Three Yin Crossing

Use this potent point for vaginal pain and itching and edema in the ankles. It is **located** approximately four finger widths above the anklebone on the inside of the leg.

Womb and Vitals

Use this very effective point to reduce lower-back pain, pain radiating from the hips, and for sciatica. It is **located** about two finger widths from the large bone at the base of the spine (sacrum).

Repeat this exercise three times before going on to the relaxation exercises.

Time: Approximately nine minutes.

Relaxation Exercises

Refer to day three for a description of the complete head-to-toe relaxation exercises. When you have finished the relaxation portion of today's exercises, repeat Centering Ch'i three times. Remain seated for a few moments after the last centering exercise.

Time: Approximately three minutes.

5

Acupressure's Healing Points

On a cold December morning four years ago, I slipped on some black ice on our driveway. By the time I reached a walk-in clinic, I was in excruciating pain. The X rays showed a lateral fracture a little over one-third of the distance along the femoral head of my right hip. I was able to return to work—on crutches—but unable to drive a car and restricted from many of my usual activities. My three month check-up X rays indicated that the fracture had healed and that surgery would not be required. Because the break itself had healed—something I could see for myself once the area was pointed out to me on the X ray—I felt that the orthopedist's dire predictions of pain and continuing stress on the joint were exaggerated warnings intended to prevent reinjury. I could not have been more wrong. Though there were many days during which I had no pain or trouble walking at all, from time to time, the pain came back and on those days I dragged my right leg behind me and was forced to sit and rest every few minutes.

I tried acupuncture and massage. Both of these treatments were restful and invigorating and provided temporary relief, but they could not help me in a substantial way from day to day. Because she is a shiatsu practitioner, my massage therapist uses acupressure points as part of her treatments. She recommended acupressure as a supplement to her treatments since acupressure was something that I could do myself whenever I felt the need. She introduced me to the Womb and Vitals point, which is two finger widths on either side of the large bony area at the base of the spine. Whenever I begin to feel tension or an ache across my lower back radiating from my right hip, I fist my hands against the back of the chair (for more leverage) at the Womb and Vitals point.

In addition, while researching other acupressure points to use during T'ai Chi class, I discovered the pressure point called the Commanding Middle, which is located in the middle of the crease behind the knee. The Womb and Vitals point and the Commanding Middle point are equally effective. Pressing either point while breathing deeply into the hip joint relieves the soreness after a few minutes and I'm able to continue working without limping and without pain. My hip will never be as strong as it was before the injury, but acupressure has made it possible for me to be virtually pain free every day.

What are Acupuncture and Acupressure?

Acupuncture involves the use of needles inserted at strategic points on the body. Acupressure is administered to the same points on the body but with finger pressure only. While acupuncture is certainly an effective method for balancing and healing, it requires from eight to ten years of medical training and an in-depth knowledge of anatomy and physiology. Acupressure is an effective and viable alternative because it can be self-administered quite easily and safely using only the pressure of your fingers. The pressure points are easy to learn, and you can use the points on yourself or on anyone else without having to worry about potential side effects.

Acupressure and acupuncture are the oldest medical treatments still being practiced all over the world today. Both methods of treatment began in the same country, at the same time in history and under the same peculiar set of circumstances.

Five thousand years ago, stones and arrows were the only available weapons on the battlefield. Many soldiers returned from war with remarkable stories of healing. Puncture wounds from arrows and bruises inflicted by rocks, while temporarily painful, actually seemed to have a healing effect on chronic illnesses and previous injuries. Puzzled, the Chinese doctors set to work to discover why this was so. Repeated experimentation on a variety of patients proved that the pressure of a finger or the puncture of a needle could and did consistently heal chronic illnesses and alleviate pain. These ancient Chinese doctors took their reasoning one step further. In order for the pressure points to be effective in healing, there had to be a system of interconnecting pathways throughout the body that linked the points themselves to organs, joints, and muscle groups. They called these pathways meridians.

The Meridians

The meridians, or pathways, defined in acupressure are, by necessity, less generalized and more precise than in the practice of T'ai Chi. Each of these meridians relates to one of five organs—lungs, heart, kidneys, liver, and the Conception Vessel, which includes the uterus, ovaries, fallopian tubes, and breasts. In addition, there are acupressure points along the meridians that govern one of six bowels. These bowels, as identified by the original practitioners of acupressure, are the large and small intestines, gallbladder, bladder, stomach, and spleen. The pericardium, Governing Vessel, and Extra Point are recognized as additional pressure points for treatment. Pressure on any of these specific points sends electrical impulses to the part or parts of the body to which that point is connected, reducing pain, inflammation, and disease.

Where several meridians converge at one point, more than one organ, bowel, or other internal system will be affected so acupressure points are divided into three general categories: local, tonic, and trigger. As the name implies, *local* refers to the area of the injury, pain, or weakness. Using the acupressure point nearest the affected area can strengthen the joint, muscle, or organ. Unless you have professional training in the field of acupressure, experimentation is the best way to learn what will work in each situation. Always begin with the gentlest touch.

Gradually increase the pressure if it is necessary and you feel that it is safe. Eventually, you will learn what types of acupressure to use for each part of your body. Brisk rubbing or kneading may be required to relieve pain in an overworked or stressed part of the body, particularly on large muscle groups. Light pressure should always be used if the area is sensitive to the touch. If the pressure point is on a large bone and that bone is not fractured, firm pressure is usually recommended to speed up the healing process.

The term *trigger point* refers to a point some distance away from the area of injury. You will notice as you practice acupressure that sometimes you will press on one point and feel a reaction somewhere else on your body. In that case, after you have completed your treatment of the original local point, move on to the area where you felt a response. Press on that point for an amount of time equal to that spent on the first point. The fact that you felt *referred* pain may indicate a blockage somewhere along the meridians of those two locations or at a juncture point.

Because meridians channel electrical energy to all parts of the body, there are *tonic* points along those pathways that serve to both calm and invigorate the system as a whole. These points are not related to specific organs, joints, or muscle groups but instead directly target the entire immune system, calm the spirit, and animate the flow of nourishing blood and healing lymph. Use of these points every day will help you to maintain good health throughout your life.

Acupressure can be used as I have done to control pain and strengthen the site of a serious injury and as a supplement to professional therapy. Preparing the muscles with acupressure prior to a chiropractic treatment makes the adjustments that much more effective for you and easier for your doctor. Professionally administered or self-administered acupressure will enhance professional care for even the most serious of illnesses such as asthma, diabetes, or cancer. Also, pressure points may be used simply to tone and relax muscles.

There are five types of pressure that are recommended for different points and needs:

1. *Firm* pressure for four or five seconds to stimulate a point for general relief.
2. The *gradual application* of pressure, holding the point for several minutes to relax muscles and relieve pain.
3. Slow *kneading* for large muscle groups.
4. *Brisk rubbing* to stimulate the flow of blood and lymph to a painful area.
5. For delicate areas such as the face, use quick, light *finger tapping* while a *loose fist* works better for large areas such as the pressure points on the back and buttocks.

Acupressure appears to close the gates of the pain centers in the brain, i.e., the neurons that are activated by somatosensory signals received and transmitted through the nerve endings. In addition, stimulating certain pressure points seems to trigger the release of the neurochemicals called *endorphins*. These neurochemicals have a morphinelike effect on aching joints, sore muscles, and the pain that accompanies an injury. Other neurochemicals such as norepinephrine, dopamine, and serotonin are also released during the application of acupressure. These chemical products of the brain help to balance the emotions, relax the body, and uplift the spirit. Along with the neurochemicals, pressing points along the meridians related to organs and systems increases circulation bringing nourishing blood and immune producing lymph to all parts of the body.

Points to Help Breathing

A former student of mine suffered for a number of years with various breathing problems. She used a breathing machine during the day and all night as well as three different types of inhalers. Her doctor encouraged her to go without the oxygen whenever possible, but she was unable to do so for more than a few minutes at a time. She learned deep-breathing exercises in our seated T'ai Chi class, and I showed her a few acupressure points that I felt might be helpful. She began using these points every day along with several of the breathing exercises and discovered that she was able to go without her oxygen for longer periods of time.

Breathing problems may be of long standing, such as asthma, or the problem may be due to advanced age, as was the case with the student just mentioned. Sometimes, diet and a sedentary lifestyle are at the root of these difficulties so it is always wise to analyze what you eat and resolve to become more physically active. The exercises outlined in the previous chapter or the shorter version in Chapter 5 will greatly improve your level of wellness with the emphasis on deep diaphragmatic breathing. The following acupressure points may be used in conjunction with the exercises or in addition to those outlined in the Relaxation Exercises section.

Colds and Flu

Medical research indicates that up to 80 percent of our illnesses may be due to stress. Stress reduces the body's ability to fight off infections and leaves us vulnerable to the multitude of germs to which we are exposed. Further damage ensues when we have a cold or the flu. The strain put on our upper-respiratory system by an invading virus significantly restricts our ability to oxygenate our cells properly.

Unless you have a fever, go ahead and practice your seated T'ai Chi exercises. They are gentle enough to be helpful without aggravating your illness. The deep breathing that accompanies all the exercises will help to reduce stresses brought on by a sore throat, muscle aches, and headaches. During the Relaxation Exercises section, substitute some of the following points for those that are not cold or flu specific. In between exercise sessions, use these pressure points to reduce your symptoms.

Bladder Meridian No. 2—Drilling Bamboo

Press your thumbs upward at the indentations at the ridge of the eyebrows on the inside corners of the eye sockets. Press firmly and hold for one minute.

Additional Benefits: Reduces the pain of frontal headaches and relieves tired eyes. This point also clears foggy vision, reduces the effects of hay fever by clearing the sinuses.

Stomach Meridian No. 3—Facial Beauty

Slide your fingers along your cheekbone until they are directly below the pupils of your eyes. Press upward against the left cheekbone with the middle finger of your left hand and against the right cheekbone with the middle finger of your right hand. Keep your fingers together to steady your hand and to exert firmer pressure. Hold for thirty to sixty seconds.

Additional Benefits: Repeated use of this pressure point will firm sagging cheeks and improve circulation to the skin giving you a more vibrant complexion. This point relieves head congestion, a stuffy nose and burning eyes, and clears the sinuses.

Large Intestine Meridian No. 20—Welcoming Perfume

Press your index fingers at the base of the nose, one finger on either side of the nostrils and above the lips. Do not push against the nostrils. Breathe deeply through your nose and hold for thirty to sixty seconds.

Additional Benefits: Relieves sinus pain and stuffy nose.

Large Intestine Meridian No. 11—Crooked Pond

This is a familiar pressure point since we use this during the relaxation section of the T'ai Chi exercises. Just as a reminder, this point is on the top of the arm at the end of the elbow crease. If you fold your arms, you can press on both arms at the same time. Use your middle fingers since you will be able to apply more pressure with your middle fingers than with your index fingers. Hold again for thirty to sixty seconds.

Additional Benefits: Strengthens the immune system and relieves constipation. Use of this point will alleviate the fever that sometimes accompanies

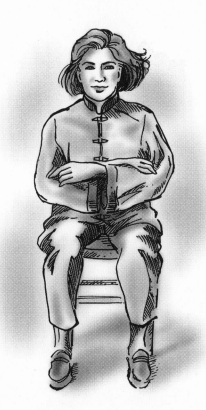

Crooked Pond

a cold and elbow pain due to arthritis while, at the same time, benefiting the immune system and stimulating the intestines.

Large Intestine Meridian No. 4—Joining the Valley

If you have already used either the long or short exercise format, you will be familiar with this pressure point as well. Press on the flap of skin between your thumb and index finger with the thumb and index finger of your other hand. Your fingers should be placed immediately in front of the joint between these two fingers.

Additional Benefits: This is an anti-inflammatory point that can be used to relieve headaches and toothaches as well as constipation. This point is also helpful for restoring health to the liver, for balancing the gastrointestinal system, and relieving feelings of depression.

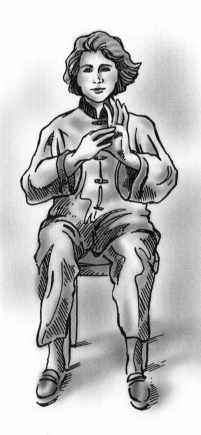

Joining the Valley

Gallbladder Meridian No. 20—Gates of Consciousness

On either side of the two large ropy muscles in your neck (trapezius) and the set of muscles that end at the mastoid bones (sternoclineidomastoid) at the base of the skull is a hollow area. Press your middle fingers on both sides and hold for thirty to sixty seconds.

Additional Benefits: Relieves irritability and reduces the pain of arthritis. This is a good pressure point to use when you are having trouble falling asleep. Use this point to relieve a stiff neck, a headache, or hypertension.

Governing Vessel Meridian No. 16—Wind Mansion

This is another point we used during our seated T'ai Chi program that many of my students have found very helpful. It is located in the hollow at the base of the skull. Press with your middle finger for thirty to sixty seconds. You should feel an immediate loosening of your sinuses.

Additional Benefits: Use this point if you have a nosebleed or are suffering from vertigo. This point will also relieve neck aches, headaches, and a sore throat as it clears the head and nose.

Governing Vessel Meridian No. 24.5—Third Eye Point

Press your index finger on the small indentation between your eyebrow at the top of your nose bone. You may remember this as the center of intuition. Hold your index finger lightly on this point and breathe deeply for thirty to sixty seconds.

Additional Benefits: This point may be used to reduce irritability, confusion, and depression. It also is a stimulant for the immune system. Use this point to relieve fatigue and for stomach disorders and nausea

Kidney Meridian No. 27—Elegant Mansion

Move your fingers along your collarbone until you feel the small hollows on either side of your breastbone. Press your fingers on those points for thirty to sixty seconds. This is an effective point to use if you have sore throat with your cold.

Additional Benefits: This point is beneficial for anxiety attacks and the hiccups. K 27 also strengthens the kidneys, the lungs, and the throat. Use this point if you have a cough.

Sinusitis and Hay Fever

There are many of us who are miserable through the entire growing season of spring and equally uncomfortable at the end of the summer. Pollens in the air cause hay fever and pet hair and dander, room fresheners, chemical cleaning solutions, and sprays may result in chronic sinusitis. Irritants that cause swelling in the ostium, which is a hairpin-shaped tube that opens into the sinuses, will block the opening to those sinuses causing a build up of mucus. Because we can't possibly avoid all the things that can cause sinusitis and hay fever, we need to find ways to relieve the worst of these symptoms. Diet plays a role in our reactions to irritants and you should consult your doctor for ways to control your symptoms.

Staying active with your seated T'ai Chi exercises and using the deep-breathing techniques outlined in Chapters 3 and 5 will help to clear your head and nasal passages. Pay close attention to your diet and avoid those foods that intensify allergic reactions. In addition, make use of the following points with your exercises or whenever you need them. The points listed in the previous section for colds and the flu are useful for sinus problems and hay fever as well.

Bladder Meridian No. 10—Heavenly Pillar

There are two large muscles at the back of your neck that rise from the shoulders and end at the base of the skull. They are called the trapezius muscles. Measure approximately two finger widths below the base of the skull on these two muscles. This is the location of Heavenly Pillar. Press with your middle finger or with your middle and index fingers held together. Breathe deeply while you hold your fingers on this point and send the energy to your head and sinus cavities.

Additional Benefits: This point is helpful to relax the entire body and overcome insomnia. Use this point if you are suffering from stress, burnout, or overexertion. Heavenly Pillar opens the sensory organs.

Bladder Meridian No. 7—Penetrate Heaven

Run your hand directly upward from the top of your ear to within one thumb width from the top of your head. Your fingers should be in a direct line with the backs of your ears. You may press on either side or both sides at the same time.

Additional Benefits: This point will improve your sense of smell if it is weak. Use this point for headaches and nasal and head congestion

Governing Vessel Meridian No. 20—One Hundred Meeting Point

This point is located where a baby's soft spot is. In line with the backs of your ears slide your finger up to the very top of your head. Press firmly for thirty to sixty seconds.

Additional Benefits: This point is recommended to improve memory and concentration as well as to relieve plugged sinuses. Use this point also for hot flashes, heatstroke, and headache.

Governing Vessel Meridian No. 26—Middle of a Person

You can find this point right below your nose at the indentation between your nose bone and your gums. To control a sneeze, press this point for thirty to sixty seconds.

Additional Benefits: If you begin to feel faint, press this point and your weakness and dizziness will pass. This point is also effective for cramps, hay fever, and to promote clearer thinking.

Chronic Breathing Problems

The Centers for Disease Control and Prevention recently issued a report that there has been an alarming increase in the last few years in the number of children with asthma. Chronic breathing problems are on the upswing with all segments of the population, though not quite to the extent found among our youngest. Diet, lifestyle, and pollutants in the air both at home and in the schools are blamed for the escalation of this debilitating condition according to the EPA.

Deep, diaphragmatic breathing is one solution to this problem along with the pressure points used in Chinese medicine. The Elegant Mansion point, which is used for colds and the flu, is helpful for chronic conditions also. The following four points are helpful to prevent or reduce the symptoms of asthma and other breathing difficulties.

Bladder Meridian No. 13—Lung Associated Point

This point is difficult to use effectively on yourself. You will probably need someone else to help you. The Lung Associated Point can be found between the spine and the scapula. Measure one finger width below the upper tip of the shoulder blade. Press and hold for at least one minute.

Additional Benefits: This point may be used to relieve muscle spasms in the neck and shoulders as well as for breathing difficulties and for opening the chest.

Lung Meridian No. 1—Letting Go

You can find this pressure point on the outer part of the chest and three finger widths below the collarbone. Press your middle finger on this point for thirty to sixty seconds. Repeat as often as necessary.

Additional Benefits: Use this point for emotional upset and distress. This point is effective for asthma, fatigue, any breathing difficulties and for relieving wrist pain.

Lung Meridian No. 9—Great Abyss

There is a small indentation at the base of the thumb on the inside of the hand. Press thumb or middle finger on this point for thirty to sixty seconds.

Additional Benefits: Use to reduce anxiety and irritation. This point is effective for relieving asthma and coughing as it balances the lungs.

Lung Meridian No. 10—Fish Border

From the Great Abyss point, slide your finger up your thumb. There is a large bone where the thumb joins the index finger. Move your fingers upward from that large bone to the middle of the fleshy bulge that forms the thumb pad and inward toward your palm. Press on this point for thirty to sixty seconds.

Additional Benefits: This point will improve your ability to breathe deeply and can reduce a swollen throat. Use this point to relieve wrist pain and emotional distress as well as for asthma or any breathing difficulties.

Whole-Body Healing Points

Allergies

An allergic reaction is an excessive response of the body's immune system to invasion by a foreign substance. The most common invaders are pollens, pet hair and dander, dust, spores and molds. Allergies are so common today that drugstore shelves are filled with an endless array of pills, nasal sprays, syrups, and water-soluble tablets. It is encouraging to know that we can also alleviate allergy symptoms with exercise, deep-breathing techniques and acupressure.

Several of the students in my classes suffer from seasonal and environmental allergies. Because we have found them to be the most effective, we use the Crooked Pond point and the Valley Point every day. Though the causes of each person's discomfort may vary, these acupressure points provide the relief we all need. I now carry a box of tissues with me to class. By the end of our acupressure session, everyone's sinuses have cleared!

Large Intestine Meridian No. 11—Crooked Pond

This pressure point should be familiar to you since it is included in the relaxation portion of the exercises. In case you have forgotten, this point is on the top of the arm at the end of the elbow crease. If you wish you may stimulate this point on both arms at the same time by folding them and pressing at the end of the crease at your elbow. Or, if you prefer, hold one arm straight and, using your other hand, press at the outer end of the elbow crease. Hold for thirty to sixty seconds and then change arms.

Additional Benefits: This point is useful for stimulating the intestines thereby relieving constipation. Crooked Pond may also be pressed to reduce the pain of arthritis at the elbow joint. Use this point to reduce the fever of a cold and to benefit your immune system.

Kidney Meridian No. 27—Elegant Mansion

Find this point by sliding your finger along the collarbone to the breastbone. There is a hollow on each side of the breastbone that is the location of Elegant Mansion. Press with your middle finger on one side, or hold your fingers on both sides at the same time for at least one full minute.

Additional Benefits: Use this point if you have the hiccups. Hold for one minute. If you still have the hiccups, press and hold again. Repeat as often as necessary. This point is effective for anxiety, coughing, a sore throat, and strengthening the kidneys.

Bladder Meridian No. 10—Heavenly Pillar

At the back of your neck, there are two thick muscles (trapezius) running vertically from your shoulders to the base of the skull. Press on either or both muscles at a distance of about $\frac{1}{2}$ inch below the skull.

Additional Benefits: This is a wonderful point to use if you are feeling tired. Swelling of the eyes will be reduced if you press on this point several times a day.

Large Intestine Meridian No. 4—Joining the Valley

Do not use this point if you are pregnant. It may stimulate premature contractions. For the relief of allergies, though, press on the webbing between your thumb and index finger. Make sure that your working thumb and index finger are pressing as close to the joint between the thumb and finger of the hand you are pressing on.

Additional Benefits: This point also strengthens the liver and balances the gastrointestinal system. Use this point for the pain of frontal headaches, for constipation, and to alleviate depression.

Triple Warmer Meridian No. 5—Outer Gate

This pressure point is located two and a half finger widths below the wrist crease on the lower forearm between the two large arm bones. Press and hold on this point for thirty to sixty seconds.

Additional Benefits: You may use this point to strengthen your immune system and to reduce the inflammation of rheumatism. This point also regulates all the systems and relaxes the entire body.

Conception Vessel Meridian No. 6—Sea of Energy

Place your index finger at the bottom of your navel and measure two finger widths below it. Press firmly on this point for a full minute.

Additional Benefits: This pressure point may be used to relieve gas and constipation. It is helpful to reduce a general weakness of the system. Use this point to strengthen your lower back muscles and for impotence.

Stomach Meridian No. 36—Three Mile Point

You can find this point by measuring four finger widths below the outside of your kneecap. You will feel a large hollow in that area. Press and hold for one minute. Repeat as necessary.

Additional Benefits: This point is extremely helpful if you have indigestion or gas. Use this point also for relieving fatigue and to boost your immune system.

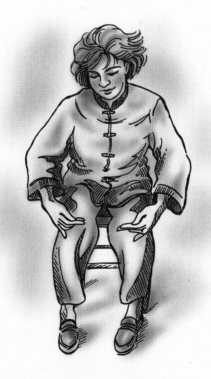

Three Mile Point

Anxiety and Nervousness

Seated T'ai Chi, with its emphasis on deep-breathing and balancing exercises, is perfectly designed to address emotional highs and lows. If you are experiencing an unusually stressful period in your life, it is important to set time aside to go through all the T'ai Chi exercises. Stress may be an unavoidable element of adulthood but it need not become the center of our lives.

There is a preventive component of both T'ai Chi and acupressure. Practicing your exercises and selecting the proper points to use for nervousness and worry may avert a full blown anxiety attack. Acupressure points such as Heavenly Pillar and the Third Eye Point are helpful to reduce anxiety. They are not found in the following list because they are included as remedies previous sections. Use the following points in conjunction with the T'ai Chi relaxation exercises. You may add one or two of these or substitute them for those you do not particularly need.

Triple Warmer Meridian No. 15—Heavenly Rejuvenation

Unless you are suffering from bursitis or stiffness of your shoulder joints, you should be able to reach this point yourself. Measure one finger width from the base of your neck. Move your finger back about $\frac{1}{2}$ inch from the shoulder at the middle of the large muscle. Remember to breathe deeply as you press this point and hold for one minute.

Additional Benefits: Use this point to eliminate the pain of a stiff neck and to reduce the recurrence of colds. Heavenly Rejuvenation is also helpful to reduce nervous tension as it calms the nerves and to relax shoulder muscles.

Pericardium Meridian No. 3—Crooked Marsh

Hold your arm straight so that the inside of the arm is facing forward. Run your finger from the outside edge of the elbow crease at the Crooked Pond point to the inside end of the elbow crease. This is the Crooked Marsh point. Press on this point with your middle finger for one minute.

Additional Benefits: Use this pressure point for pains in your arms or elbows. Crooked Marsh also relieves a nervous stomach and reduces anxiety and palpitations as it regulates the heart and balances the emotions.

Pericardium Meridian No. 6—Inner Gate

Hold your arm out straight again. Trace down your forearm to its inner side. Two and a half finger widths above the wrist crease is where you will want to put pressure. Hold your middle finger on this point for thirty to sixty seconds.

Additional Benefits: Use this point if you are experiencing pains in your wrist. This point is also helpful for relieving nausea and insomnia as it balances the internal organs and calms the spirit.

Heart Meridian No. 7—Spirit Gate

This point is located on the outside of the forearm (little finger side) at the crease of the wrist. Use your other thumb or middle finger and hold for thirty to sixty seconds.

Additional Benefits: This point will reduce incidence of forgetfulness, strengthen the heart and uplift your spirits. Use this point for insomnia caused by overexcitement and to relieve anxiety.

Conception Vessel Meridian No. 17—Sea of Tranquillity

Trace down the middle of your breastbone with your finger to the base of the bone and then measure three thumb widths up. This is a very useful pressure point for many emotional disturbances. Press strongly on this point with your middle finger for one minute.

Additional Benefits: Use this point to get rid of the blues as well as for more severe types of depression. This point balances the emotions as it calms the spirit.

Arthritis

Osteoarthritis is the most common form of arthritis and is prevalent among people age 55 and older. This is characterized by the breakdown of the cartilage cushion in joints. Inflammatory arthritis is characterized by an inflammation of the joints and tendons. Joints may appear red and warm to the touch because chemicals released in the tissue surrounding the joint increase blood flow to that area. Because of the pain associated with inflammation, people who suffer from this type of arthritis will usually avoid using the affected joint. After a period of time, immobilizing these joints to lessen the pain stiffens the tendons and tightens the muscles surrounding the inflamed joint. If this condition persists, the joints may bow out or curl under until there is no mobility at all.

Most, if not all, physicians recommend regular exercise of the low-impact variety to help arthritis. Seated T'ai Chi is ideal for people with either of these forms of arthritis. Additional help can be found in acupressure. Certain points are especially effective to reduce the inflammation and pain of arthritis. Use of these pressure points during the relaxation period of the exercises in addition to, or in place of, others will greatly relieve the symptoms of pain and swelling.

Large Intestine Meridian No. 11—Crooked Pond

This is a multipurpose pressure point that is located at the upper end of the elbow crease. By folding your arms, you will be able to press the point on each elbow at the same time if you wish. Otherwise, hold your arm out straight or bend it to your chest and, using your index finger, apply pressure strongly and hold for a full minute. Don't forget to breathe into the targeted area.

Additional Benefits: By stimulating the intestines, this point will relieve constipation and balance the immune system at the same time. Use this point also for relieving the fever of a cold and for arthritis pain in the elbow.

Gallbladder Meridian No. 20—Gates of Consciousness

You can find this pressure point in the hollows at the base of the skull. There are two large muscles extending upward from the shoulders called the trapezius muscles. Between these two muscles and your ears is another set of slightly smaller muscles called the sternoclineidomastoids. Between these two sets of muscles is a large hollow. Press on these hollows for thirty to sixty seconds.

Additional Benefits: Use this point if you have a headache or are having difficulty falling asleep. Gates of Consciousness is also effective for a stiff neck and for hypertension.

Triple Warmer Meridian No. 5—Outer Gate

Between the two bones of the forearm above the wrist crease is where the Outer Gate is located. Measure two and a half finger widths from the wrist crease on the inside of your arm. Your pressing finger will be slightly more toward the outside of the arm than the inside. Hold for thirty to sixty seconds.

Additional Benefits: This point is also useful for allergic reactions, rheumatism, and tendonitis. Use this point also to regulate and relax your whole body.

Stomach Meridian 36—Three Mile Point

Measure four finger widths below your kneecap on the outside of the leg. You will find a good-sized hollow between the bones. Press on the this point and hold for one minute breathing in to the area as you do so.

Additional Benefits: This point is very effective for indigestion, nausea, and gas. Use the Three Mile Point for fatigue and to rebuild your immune system.

Chronic Fatigue Syndrome

The existence of this disease came to the public's attention in the 1980s. Though there is still some controversy surrounding the exact cause of this illness, it is generally believed to be a virus that attacks the immune system during times of prolonged stress. The virus may have been present but dormant for many years before the onset of the disease. It does appear, however, that the trigger is stress. Stress over a period of time weakens the immune system and allows the virus to overtake the body's defense mechanism.

Use the following pressure points to relieve ordinary fatigue. If you have been diagnosed with chronic fatigue syndrome, the process may take several months with at least three applications per day before you begin to feel the effects.

Liver Meridian No. 3—Bigger Rushing

You will find this pressure point on the top of your foot between the big toe and the second toe. Press and hold for one minute.

Additional Benefits: Use this point for dizziness as well as fatigue and for headaches and nausea. Bigger Rushing is also helpful for arthritis pain, tired eyes, nasal congestion, and hangovers. This point invigorates and clears all the systems of your body.

Pericardium Meridian No. 6—Inner Gate

Between the two large bones of your forearm on the inside of the arm lies the Inner Gate point. Measure two and a half finger widths from the wrist. Press on this point for one minute.

Additional Benefits: This is an effective point for relief from nausea and wrist pain. Also use this point to relieve indigestion and to balance all the internal organs.

Lung Meridian No. 1—Letting Go

Find this point on your outer chest about four finger widths above the armpit. Measure one finger width inward from the shoulder bone. Press and hold for one minute.

Additional Benefits: Use this point for coughing, asthma, and to control excessive emotions. This point is also helpful for relieving confusion and irritability as well as for strengthening the lungs.

Bladder Meridian Nos. 23 and 47—Sea of Vitality

You can find this pressure point in the lower part of your back at waist level. Measure four finger widths from the spine. Use light pressure only if you have back problems. You will need to use both hands fisted at this point, or have someone else press the point for you. If you prefer to use a firmer pressure and have no one to press on this point for you, sit in a chair, place your hands on this point between your back and the back of the chair. Lean into your hands for one minute.

Additional Benefits: This is an effective point for relieving backaches and impotence. Use this point to strengthen your kidneys and immune system, to relieve fatigue and to strengthen your digestive organs.

Gallbladder Meridian No. 21—Shoulder Well

To find this point, slide your finger from the base of your neck one to two finger widths along the large muscle of the shoulder. Press and hold for one full minute. If you are pregnant, press very lightly and reduce the amount of time to no more than thirty seconds.

Additional Benefits: If your hands or feet are cold, press on this point to stimulate the circulation to your limbs. This is also an effective pressure point to relieve the pain of a headache, to decrease feelings of nervousness, irritability, fatigue, and shoulder pain. This point softens any hard, tense muscles.

Governing Vessel Meridian No. 24.5—Third Eye Point

This point is located between your eyebrows and between the base of your forehead and the top of your nose bone. Press and hold for one minute.

Additional Benefits: The Third Eye Point is an excellent pressure point to use for relieving headaches and alleviating depression. This point also relieves glandular imbalances, irritability, depression, and confusion as well as stimulating the immune system.

Constipation

Most people have to deal with constipation at some time in their lives. Four factors contribute to occasional constipation: diet, stress, lack of exercise, and dehydration. Most of us are aware that there are deficiencies in our diets, stress in our lives, and that we don't get enough exercise. Fresh fruits and vegetables, whole grains, and a well-rounded diet that includes a variety of foods from all the food groups is important to avoid being constipated.

Exercise is essential to flush toxins from the body both through the sweat glands and through the excretory system. In addition, flushing toxins will balance the body to promote good health and to maintain the proper weight. The seated T'ai Chi exercises in this book are designed to open the pathways of the body to boost the flow of energy. The energy you receive each time you practice your T'ai Chi exercises will encourage you to be more active in other facets of your life such as using the stairs instead of taking the elevator and walking rather than driving whenever possible. Since all of these exercises relax the body and calm the emotions, stress levels will be significantly reduced.

Few people recognize when they are dehydrated since there are no easily identifiable symptoms except in the rare case of severe dehydration, which generally requires hospitalization. Since the human body is made up of 25 percent solid matter and 75 percent water, optimum health is dependent on continuous rehydration just to maintain the balance between solids and fluids. An adult weighing up to 200 pounds should ideally be drinking a gallon of water per day. If you weigh over 200 pounds, an additional 8-ounce glass of water for every 10 pounds over 200 pounds is necessary to prevent dehydration. A person weighing 220 pounds, then, would have to drink a gallon plus 16 additional ounces to be fully hydrated.

Too many popular drinks contain caffeine. What do you reach for when you're thirsty? For most people, the answer would be a soft drink. Many adults carry coffee with them wherever they go. Unfortunately, although all caffeinated drinks do contain water, the caffeine in the mixture counteracts much of the effect of that water. When we drink coffee and colas, the water reserves in our bodies become severely depleted. There is not enough fluid in the system to flush waste material through the colon and out, so these materials become trapped in the intestines resulting in constipation.

For the temporary relief of constipation certain pressure points are effective. Many of these same points have been described in other sections of this chapter. If you need to refresh your memory with regard to their locations, see the following list.

Large Intestine Meridian No. 11—Crooked Pond

Bend your left arm toward your chest. Find the end of your elbow crease at the top of your arm. Press on this spot with the index finger of your left hand for one minute. Repeat several times during the day.

Additional Benefits: Use this point for arthritis pain in your elbow. This is an effective point to relieve constipation and the fever of a cold. Crooked Pond stimulates the intestines and the immune system.

Large Intestine Meridian No. 4—Joining the Valley

If you are not pregnant this is a most effective point to use for relieving constipation. Pinch your index finger and thumb against the flap of skin between the same two fingers of your other hand at the point where the bones of the index finger and the thumb meet. Hold for one minute.

Additional Benefits: This point is useful for toothaches and arthritis in the hand, wrist, elbow, shoulder, and neck. Use this point also for frontal headaches, constipation, and depression.

Conception Vessel Meridian No. 6—Sea of Energy

Measure three finger widths below your navel. Press firmly on this point for one minute. Repeat as often as necessary.

Additional Benefits: This is an effective pressure point for strengthening the lower back as it energizes the entire body. You may also find this point helpful to relieve constipation and gas.

Stomach Meridian No. 36—Three Mile Point

Place your index finger at the outside edge of your kneecap. Where your little finger touches against the leg, you will feel a depression. Press on one or both legs at this point with your middle finger. Hold for one minute.

Additional Benefits: Use this point if you are feeling tired or if you have had a recent bout with the flu. This point is also effective for stomach disorder and nausea and to restore the immune system.

Fainting

The following acupressure points may be used for occasional fainting spells brought on by going without meals, periods of extreme excitement, or a generally weakened system. Use these pressure points on yourself when you first begin to feel faint. If you faint frequently, however, see your physician.

Liver Meridian No. 3—Bigger Rushing

Press on the area between your big toe and second toe in the depression between the two bones. Hold for one minute. Repeat if you are still feeling weak.

Additional Benefits: Use this point if you have a hangover. In addition, this point is helpful for the pain of arthritis, headaches, tired eyes, nasal congestion, and to invigorate the entire system.

Kidney Meridian No. 1—Bubbling Spring

You can find this point on the ball of your foot between the pad directly below the big toe and the pad that runs underneath the other toes. Press firmly for one minute.

Additional Benefits: This pressure point may be used for convulsions and hot flashes. Use this point for impotence and to stimulate the kidneys.

Governing Vessel Meridian No. 26—Middle of a Person

This point is located at the base of the nose between the nose bone and the upper ridge of the gums. Press and hold firmly for one minute.

Additional Benefits: Use this point for cramps, moments of extreme emotional distress, or pain along the spine. This point is also helpful for dizziness and hay fever.

Hot Flashes

If you have ever experienced hot flashes you don't need a medical definition to recognize the symptoms. During menopause, estrogen levels decrease causing the area of the brain that regulates body temperature to receive the wrong signals. Elevated levels of norepinephrine stimulate the brain mechanism that is the body's thermostat.

Hot flashes usually begin at the waist or chest and move upward to the neck and head. They occur most frequently in the evening or during hot weather. It is possible to suffer an episode as often as every hour and a half. Most of these episodes last anywhere from fifteen seconds to half an hour. The average time experienced by most menopausal women, however, is five minutes.

A lighter diet, lighter clothes, and cool drinks will help to reduce your body temperature. Use the pressure points below to reduce the occurrence and severity of the episodes.

Kidney Meridian No. 1—Bubbling Spring

Locate this pressure point, place your hand on the ball of your foot. Between the two pads that make up the ball, press your thumb and hold for one minute.

Additional Benefits: Use this pressure point to prevent fainting. This point stimulates the kidneys and rejuvenates the spirit.

Governing Vessel Meridian No. 20—One Hundred Meeting Point

This point is on the crown of the head where the soft spot is on babies. Trace a line from the backs of your ears to the very top of your head. Press and hold on this point for one minute.

Additional Benefits: This point is effective for heatstroke and to improve memory and concentration. Use this point also for headaches and to calm the emotions.

Conception Vessel No. 17—Sea of Tranquillity

You can find this pressure point in the middle of your breastbone. Measure three thumb widths above the solar plexus, i.e., above the base of the breastbone. Use your middle finger to press firmly on this point for one minute.

Additional Benefits: Use this point if you have insomnia or are depressed. The Sea of Tranquillity point balances the emotions and calms the spirit.

Upper-Body Healing Points

Kathleen had been experiencing stomach cramps and nausea for an hour after eating in a restaurant. She said the food was a bit greasy and the meat wasn't cooked as thoroughly as it should have been. I suggested that she try the Three Mile Point for one minute several times during the day and drink several glasses of warm or lukewarm water. Within just a few hours, her cramps were gone and she was no longer feeling nauseated.

Relief for stomachaches and toothaches will be addressed in this section along with helpful centers for reducing neck pain and skin problems such as acne and eczema. All of the acupressure points described here target problems you may experience with your ears, eyes, head or jaw including points to improve your concentration and memory. Topics are listed in alphabetical order for your convenience. Many of these point will be familiar to you from the previous two sections because every acupressure point results in multiple benefits for various parts of the body.

Earaches

The following pressure points are intended for use in cases of common earache from viral infections or a cold. If you fly in airplane and the takeoff and landings are a problem for you, the points listed in this section will be very helpful. If you have a history of ear pain or blockage, there may be a more serious underlying medical cause for which you should consult your physician.

Kidney Meridian No. 3—Bigger Stream

This point is located on your ankle halfway between your ankle bone and the Achilles' tendon. Press and hold for one minute.

Additional Benefits: Use this point for painful wisdom teeth. This point restores health to the reproductive system and stimulates the immune system. Fatigue, swollen feet, and insomnia all benefit from the use of this pressure point as well.

Gallbladder Meridian No. 2—Reunion of Hearing
Small Intestine Meridian No. 19—Listening Place
Triple Warmer Meridian No. 21—Ear Gate

All three of these points are directly in front of your ear. Open your mouth and you will notice that there is a deep depression caused by the lowering of your jaw. Listening Place is directly in front of the ear opening while Ear Gate is $\frac{1}{2}$ inch above and Reunion of Hearing is $\frac{1}{2}$ inch below. Your mouth should still be partly open while you press on all three locations at the same time. Hold for at least five minutes or until you begin to feel relief.

Additional Benefits: These points are helpful for relief from headaches and for balancing the thyroid gland. Use these pressure points also for water in the ear, to open a plugged ear, and to relieve the pain of TMJ problems.

Triple Warmer Meridian No. 17—Windscreen

Run your finger upward from the angle of your jawbone to the back of your earlobe where there is a hollow spot. Press your finger lightly at this point and hold for thirty to sixty seconds or longer if you are not immediately relieved.

Additional Benefits: Use this point to relieve to clear up acne, jaw pain, sore throats, and to relieve tense facial muscles.

Eye Strain

Any time you spend too long in front of a computer or TV screen, your eyes are apt to become tired and strained. Take a minute, close your eyes, and use the following acupressure points to relieve your eyes whether they are red or just tired or when your vision begins to blur.

Bladder Meridian No. 2—Drilling Bamboo

At the inside corner of your eyebrows where the nose bone and eye socket bone meet, press upward with your thumbs and hold for one minute while breathing deeply in through your nose and out through your mouth. Expand your diaphragm and relax.

Additional Benefits: This point is helpful for headaches and hay fever. Use this point to clear your sinuses and brighten your eyes.

Stomach Meridian No. 3—Facial Beauty

Directly below the pupil of the eye on the cheekbone is the pressure point called Facial Beauty. Close your eyes and press firmly with your index fingers on these points. Hold for one minute. Repeat as often as necessary.

Additional Benefits: You will find this point beneficial for improving your complexion and stimulating circulation to the face. You may also use this point effectively to clear head congestion, stuffy nose, and burning eyes.

Stomach Meridian No. 2—Four Whites

You will find this pressure point in the center of the bony ridge under the eye (the lowest part of the eye socket). There is a small indentation at the middle of this bone. Press your index fingers on this point on either side of your nose. Hold with a light touch for one minute.

Additional Benefits: Use this point for acne and to clear your sinuses. This pressure point also relieves burning eyes and relaxes the muscles of the eyes and face.

Bladder Meridian No. 10—Heavenly Pillar

Run your finger up your neck along the muscle closest to the spine (trapezius muscles). Press on the point that is $\frac{1}{2}$ inch from the base of the skull. Hold for one minute.

Additional Benefits: If you are having difficulty falling asleep use this point. Heavenly Pillar is also helpful for relieving stress, anxiety, burnout, and overexertion as it relaxes the entire body.

Governing Vessel Meridian No. 24.5—Third Eye Point

Press on the small indentation between your eyebrows at the top of the nose bone. Hold for one minute with your eyes closed. Breathe deeply.

Additional Benefits: This is a multipurpose pressure point. It is helpful for hay fever and headaches. Pressure on the Third Eye Point is beneficial for the endocrine system and the pituitary gland. If you are feeling irritable, depressed, or you are experiencing mental confusion, use this point to relieve the effects of these emotions.

Governing Vessel Meridian No. 16—Wind Mansion

The Wind Mansion point is in the large hollow at the base of the skull at the top of the spinal column. Press and hold for thirty to sixty seconds.

Additional Benefits: Use this point any time your sinuses are clogged or painful. This pressure point is effective also for neck aches, headaches, nose bleed, and sore throats.

Headaches

The following is a list of the most common causes of headaches:

1. The spine is out of alignment.
2. You have an allergic reaction to an irritant such as pet hair or room fresheners.
3. Your diet has not included enough fresh vegetables, fruits, and whole grains.
4. You have not been drinking enough water.
5. You may have been exposed to toxic chemicals in cleaning products.
6. Headaches often occur due to the hormonal changes of the menstrual cycle.
7. Stress.

If you suspect that your spine is out of alignment, press the Heavenly Pillar points while lying down to ensure that you are reaching deep into the muscles. Stress and tension, however, are most often the culprits behind a headache. Remember, in the Chinese view, emotional and spiritual disturbances are more often at the root of physical discomfort than any other external or any internal factors. Assess your condition as objectively as you can by reaching beyond the obvious physical stresses. In the meantime, use the following pressure points.

Gallbladder Meridian No. 41—Above Tears

This point is located on top of the foot between the fourth and fifth toes. Press your index finger one finger width from the end of the webbing between the toes. Hold for one minute.

Additional Benefits: This point is helpful for relieving hip pain and sciatica. Use this point also for water retention, headaches, sideaches, and arthritis pain.

Bladder Meridian No. 2—Drilling Bamboo

Locate the point where the eyebrow ridge meets the nose bone just below the inside corner of the eyebrows. Press your thumbs on the small indentations on each side and hold for one minute. Repeat as often as necessary.

Additional Benefits: Use this pressure point to relieve sinus congestion and clear blurred vision. Drilling Bamboo will clear sinuses and brighten your eyes.

Stomach Meridian No. 3—Facial Beauty

Run your finger along the base of your cheekbone until it is positioned directly below the pupil of your eye. Press and hold for one minute or until you feel relief.

Additional Benefits: Use this point to revitalize you complexion and reduce the appearance of sagging in the lower half of the face. This pressure point also clears head congestion, a stuffy nose, and relieves burning eyes from allergic reactions or overuse.

Gallbladder Meridian No. 20—Gates of Consciousness

Use your fingers to find the two large muscles in your neck (trapezius). Between these two muscles and another set of fairly large muscles (sternoclineidomastoids) that run underneath the mastoid bones at the base of the skull is the pressure point, Gates of Consciousness. Press both sides with your middle fingers. Hold for one to three minutes.

Additional Benefits: This point is beneficial for relieving dizziness and feelings of irritability. Use this point also for a stiff neck, headaches, neck aches, insomnia, and hypertension.

Large Intestine Meridian No. 4—Joining the Valley

Using your thumb and index finger, press on the large muscle between the thumb and index finger of your other hand as close as possible to the area where the two bones meet. Hold for at least one minute. Do not use this point if you are pregnant.

Additional Benefits: This is a particularly potent point for balancing the gastrointestinal system. Use this pressure point also for frontal headaches, constipation, depression, and to alleviate pain throughout the body.

Jaw Discomfort

The most common cause of jaw pain is the habit of clenching or grinding the teeth during sleep. There may be arthritis in the temporomandibular joint as well. The following acupressure points will help to alleviate the discomfort of pain and swelling and may be used for arthritis in conjunction with standard medical treatments for this disease.

Triple Warmer Meridian No. 21—Ear Gate
Small Intestine Meridian No. 19—Listening Place
Gallbladder Meridian No. 2—Reunion of Hearing

Place your index, middle, and ring fingers in front of your ear so that your middle finger is directly in front of the ear opening. Hold your mouth partially open as you press and hold for one minute.

Additional Benefits: Use these three points together for earaches, toothaches, and headaches. These three points balance the thyroid gland and improve hearing.

Stomach Meridian No. 6—Jaw Chariot

To find this pressure point, clench your back teeth together. Press at the point where the muscle is bulging between the upper and lower jaw. Rest your fingers against the side of your face for support as you press firmly with your middle finger on the masseter muscle.

Additional Benefits: Use this point for effective relief from a toothache or a sore throat. This pressure point is helpful to relieve stress.

Triple Warmer Meridian No. 17—Windscreen

There is a large hollow behind the lower jaw and at the bottom of your earlobe. Press lightly on this point for thirty to sixty seconds. Repeat as often as necessary.

Additional Benefits: This point is effective for the treatment of facial paralysis. Use this point also if you have acne, jaw problems, a sore throat, or ear pain.

Memory and Concentration

Aside from diagnosable medical conditions such as dementia or Alzheimer's disease, lack of concentration and a poor memory are easily addressed. Diets high in sugars and carbohydrates are thought to contribute to the inability to concentrate. Stress and emotional distress may temporarily impair thought processes and memory. Medications may be at the root of temporary or permanent memory loss, particularly among the elderly.

In addition to dietary adjustments and the avoidance of stressful situations whenever possible, the following acupressure points can clear the system and restore circulation to the brain. Use these points when you are stressed or tired.

Liver Meridian No. 3—Bigger Rushing

This pressure point is on the top of the foot between the big toe and the second toe. Press and hold for one minute.

Additional Benefits: Use this point to relieve tired eyes and reduce the effects of a hangover. This is also an effective pressure point for arthritis, headaches, and nasal congestion.

Governing Vessel Meridian No. 26—Middle of a Person

Press your index finger at the base of the nose on the top of the gum ridge. Hold for one minute.

Additional Benefits: This is an effective point to use if you feel faint or dizzy. This is also a helpful pressure point for hot flashes, heatstroke, headaches, and is beneficial for improving your memory and concentration.

Governing Vessel Meridian No. 20—One Hundred Meeting Point

This acupressure point is located on the top of the head where a baby's soft spot is. There will be a slight hollow directly upward from the backs of the ears. Press and hold for one minute.

Additional Benefits: Use this point for heatstroke, headaches, epilepsy, and to relieve hot flashes. Because this point clears the brain and calms the spirit, it is most effective for improving memory and concentration.

Conception Vessel Meridian No. 17—Sea of Tranquillity

To find this point, trace a line up the middle of your breastbone three finger widths from its base. Press firmly with your middle finger and hold for one minute.

Additional Benefits: This is an effective point for all emotional disturbances. Use this point if you are nervous or suffering from depression, grief, or any emotional trauma.

Extra Meridian Point—Sun Point

Measure half an inch from the outside edge of your eyebrows in the hollow of your temples. Press lightly for thirty to sixty seconds.

Additional Benefits: Use this point for headaches and dizziness. This is an effective point to improve your memory and to brighten your eyes.

Governing Vessel Meridian No. 24.5—Third Eye Point

This point is located between the eyebrows at the top of the nose bone. There is a small indentation where you will press with your middle or index finger. Hold for one minute.

Additional Benefits: This is considered by the Chinese to be the intuitive center. It is helpful to use this point if you are working on a creative project. This pressure point relieves glandular imbalances while it boosts your immune system and relieves irritability, depression, and confusion.

Neck Pain

In Chinese medicine, the neck is considered the physical connecting point between the body and the mind. If body and mind are at odds, this disparity will manifest itself in the neck. If you have not been in a car accident or suffered some other type of injury, do a bit of self-analysis. What is it that your mind wishes to do but your body does not or, conversely, what will satisfy the body but is not acceptable to the mind? The following acupressure points will ease the pain of a sore and stiff neck, but the underlying cause must be addressed as well.

Bladder Meridian No. 2—Drilling Bamboo

Press at the point between the bridge of the nose and the lower ridge of the eyebrows. Use your thumbs and press upward on either side of your nose for a full minute. Repeat as necessary.

Additional Benefits: This is an effective point for sinus trouble, hay fever, and tired eyes. Use this point if you are experiencing foggy vision or your eyes are dull and bloodshot.

Gallbladder Meridian No. 20—Gates of Consciousness

With your hands resting on your head, press your thumbs between the two large sets of muscles in the back of the neck on either side of the spine. Push upward toward the base of the skull for one minute.

Additional Benefits: Use this point when you have trouble falling asleep. This is an equally effective point for the relief of neck and head pain, a stiff neck, or hypertension.

Bladder Meridian No. 10—Heavenly Pillar

Find the two large muscles at the back of your neck closest to the spine (the trapezius muscles). Measure ½ inch from the base of the skull. Hold your middle fingers on the inside edge of each muscle for one full minute. Bend your neck gently to your chest then back to the center and from side to side several times. If your neck is still stiff, press again for another minute and then repeat the light neck stretches.

Additional Benefits: This point may be used to relieve anxiety and insomnia. Use this point also for burnout, overexertion, and stress.

Gallbladder Meridian No. 21—Shoulder Well

Press on the large muscle at the top of the shoulder about one to two finger widths from the base of the neck. If you are pregnant, press lightly. Otherwise, press firmly with your middle fingers on both sides and hold for one minute.

Additional Benefits: Use this pressure joint to increase circulation and reduce feelings of irritability. If your muscles are hard and tense, this point is effective for softening and relaxing.

Triple Warmer Meridian No. 16—Window of Heaven

You can find this point behind the ears in a small depression at the base of the skull approximately one finger width from the back of the ear. Press on both indentations with your middle fingers and hold for thirty to sixty seconds.

Additional Benefits: Use also if you have a headache, a stiff neck, or shoulder pain.

Governing Vessel Meridian No. 16—Wind Mansion

There is a large hollow at the base of the skull at the top of the spinal column. Press firmly with your middle finger and hold for one minute.

Additional Benefits: This pressure point is beneficial for vertigo but is also very effective for relieving sinus pressure and clearing your nose. Use this point also for neck aches, headaches, nose bleeds, and sore throats.

Skin Problems

Many skin problems are exacerbated by nervous tension and stress. Acupressure relieves stress expressed in the tightening of muscles and strain that may appear on facial skin in the form of sagging, poor color (due to decreased circulation), blotches, or pimples. Emotional distress may cause blockages in the pathways or juncture points. Pressure applied to the proper acupressure points will release the blockage, allowing the blood to circulate more freely and energy to increase to all parts of the body.

Eczema is usually attributed to food allergies. Visit your physician to find out what kinds of food are causing or aggravating your condition. Use the following points to relieve the skin patches and itching of eczema. These points will also improve your complexion and tone the facial muscles.

Stomach Meridian No. 3—Facial Beauty

Run your finger along your cheekbone until your fingers are directly below the pupils of your eyes. Press firmly at the bottom of the bone for one minute. Repeat as often as necessary.

Additional Benefits: This pressure point is particularly effective for clearing nasal congestion and tired, sore eyes. Use this point also to clear foggy vision.

Stomach Meridian No. 2—Four Whites

This point is located directly below the iris of the eye on the bottom ridge of the eye socket. You will find small indentations on each ridge. Place your middle fingers directly on the indentations and hold for thirty to sixty seconds.

Additional Benefits: Use this point for irritated eyes and for facial tension. This pressure point is also beneficial for acne, other facial blemishes, and to relax tense muscles of your face and eyes.

Bladder Meridian Nos. 23 and 47—Sea of Vitality

These two points are very close together in the lower back at waist level. For B 23, measure two finger widths from the spine. B 47 is four finger widths from the spinal column. If you have had back surgery or have any disease of the discs, consult your physician before using these points.

Additional Benefits: Use these points for backaches and to heal bruises anywhere on the body more quickly. This point is effective to improve digestion, strengthen the kidneys, and stimulate the immune system.

Stomach Meridian No. 36—Three Mile Point

Place your fingers, index through little finger, vertically along the outside of your leg. Your little finger will be touching a good-sized depression. Press on both legs at this point with your middle finger. Keep your ring and index fingers close to the middle fingers to more leverage. Hold for one minute.

Additional Benefits: This point relieves gas, indigestion, and bloating. Use this point to relieve fatigue and to restore the immune system.

Triple Warmer Meridian 17—Windscreen

Directly behind each of your ear lobes is an indentation just below the mastoid process. Press your middle fingers on each side and hold for thirty to sixty seconds.

Additional Benefits: This point is effective for the relief of the swelling and itching of hives. Use this point also if you have acne, jaw problems, a sore throat, or ear pain.

Stomachaches

Diets too high in fats and sugars, hurried meals, general stress, too many cups of coffee, and too little water are all common factors that contribute to chronic indigestion, gas, and bloating. An additional component of stomach distress according to Chinese medical practitioners is the ingestion of cold food or drinks. An extreme temperature can paralyze the stomach muscles making it impossible to complete the digestive process. Though it is tempting to drink cold beverages in hot weather, they may cause stomach pain and bloating. Cool to lukewarm drinks are advised. What should be sought is balance not the extremes of hot and cold.

If your lunch hour is always rushed, try eating less. Drink a cool, but not cold, glass of water before your meal. Remember that water is necessary for all cellular processes. It will clear your stomach and aid in the digestive process. In addition, you will feel fuller so a smaller meal will be equally satisfying. Your stomach won't have to work so hard to digest a heavy meal and you will have more time to eat slowly and chew your food thoroughly.

Conception Vessel Meridian No. 12—Center of Power

This point is located halfway between the base of the breastbone and the navel. Press firmly and deeply but hold your finger at this point no longer than two minutes at any one time. If you have a serious illness, avoid this pressure point.

Additional Benefits: This point is beneficial for headaches and constipation. If you are frustrated or experiencing emotional stress, use this point as often as necessary.

Spleen Meridian No. 4—Grandfather Grandson

You will find this point one thumb width behind the ball of the foot on the arch. Press firmly and hold for one minute.

Additional Benefits: Use this point for diarrhea and menstrual cramps. This pressure point regulates and strengthens the digestive system and will relieve feelings of anxiety.

Conception Vessel Meridian No. 6—Sea of Energy

This point is two finger widths below your belly button. Press deeply and hold for one minute. Breathe deeply and relax.

Additional Benefits: This is an effective point for the relief of lower-back pain. Use this point also for constipation and gas. If you are tired, this point is effective to replenish your energy reserves.

Toothaches

Toothaches are generally caused by cavities or gum disease. See your dentist as soon as possible. In the meantime, to relieve toothaches, use the following pressure points.

Stomach Meridian No. 3—Facial Beauty

With your fingers, trace along the bottom of your cheekbone until your fingers are directly below the pupils of your eyes. Press firmly and hold for one minute.

Additional Benefits: This point will increase circulation to the face improving the complexion. Use this point also for relieving head congestion, stuffy nose, or burning eyes.

Stomach Meridian No. 6—Jaw Chariot

To find this pressure point, clench your teeth. Find the center of the muscle between your upper and lower jaw directly in front of your earlobe. Press firmly for one minute. Repeat as often as necessary.

Additional Benefits: Use this point for jaw pain and sore throats. This pressure point is also useful for stress and toothaches.

Large Intestine Meridian No. 4—Joining the Valley

Do not use this point if you are pregnant. Press with your index finger and thumb on the large muscle in front of the joint that joins the thumb and index finger of your other hand. Press firmly and hold for one minute. This point on either hand may be used.

Additional Benefits: This is an effective point for headaches, constipation, and depression. Use this point to balance your gastrointestinal system.

Triple Warmer Meridian No. 13—Shoulder Meeting Point

Measure two finger widths below the shoulder on the outer part of the arm. Find your deltoid muscle and measure one thumb width behind it. Press firmly with your middle finger and hold for one minute. Breathe deeply and repeat as needed.

Additional Benefits: Use this point for shoulder, elbow, and arm pain as well as for toothaches. This is also an effective point for relieving headaches.

Lower-Body Healing Points

Since my fall on the ice, I frequently experience pain that radiates from my injured hip across my lower back. The two acupressure points that I use the most often to relieve pain and strengthen my lower back muscles are the Commanding Middle point and the Womb and Vitals point. A student of mine has a similar problem with chronic pain. In her case, the pain and weakness is in one of her knees. She uses the Commanding Middle point also, then the Calf's Nose point to reduce the soreness and to fortify the muscles surrounding the knee. Whether the problem is aching joints and cramps in the legs or feet, lower backache or sciatica, menstrual cramps, or diarrhea, there are pressure points in this section to help relieve the pain and discomfort.

The first set of points are intended to relieve pain and strengthen ankles and knees. These joints are subjected to constant stress. While certain types of chronic pain will need to be addressed with the help of your physician, the acupressure points described in this section are an effective method of temporary relief and a beneficial supplement to the protocol that may be recommended by your doctor.

Other pressure points explained in this section are helpful for premenstrual cramps and bloating. Careful attention to diet, increased intake of fluids (without caffeine), and exercise will all counteract the misery that sometimes accompanies the menstrual cycle. In addition, use of the appropriate points just prior to the onset of menstruation will prevent the more severe symptoms.

Cramping particularly in the legs and feet is caused by muscular tension and is often accompanied by painful spasms. Diet may be a contributing factor to repeated incidents of cramping of the feet or legs, but the overuse of certain sets of muscles virtually guarantees the onset of spasms in the area that has been overworked. Use the acupressure points for immediate relief. To avoid a recurrence of cramps and spasms, try reducing the exercises or activities that seem to be causing pain, drink plenty of water to clear the system of toxins, and analyze your dietary habits.

An incorrect diet, stress, or a viral infection can all cause diarrhea. If the diarrhea is severe, there is a danger of serious dehydration. In that case, consult your physician immediately. However, if you suffer from diarrhea only occasionally, use the acupressure points in this section to tone the abdominal muscles and rebalance the digestive system.

This section also contains a description of acupressure points that are effective for the relief of back pain and sciatica. These points will reduce the temporary soreness caused by fatigue, poor posture or stress by relaxing the muscles surrounding the painful area. Although sciatica is not the same as a lower backache it may be difficult to tell the difference Sciatica is characterized by pain that is not limited to the lower back but is felt all the way down the leg and into the foot. The sciatic nerve may be pinched between vertebrae, or a disk may be bulging out of place. If you suspect that this is the case, you will need to consult your chiropractor or physician.

Ankles and Feet

Kidney Meridian No. 3—Bigger Stream

You can find this pressure point at the hollow directly between, and in line with, the inside ankle bone and the Achilles' tendon. Press and hold for one minute. Do not use this point if you are pregnant.

Additional Benefits: Use this point for menstrual cramps, headaches, and hangovers. If you have swollen feet or you are particularly tired, this pressure point will be helpful.

Bladder Meridian No. 62—Calm Sleep

Measure one thumb width below the inside ankle bone. Bend your leg so that it is resting on the thigh or your other leg and press with your middle finger or thumb for one minute.

Additional Benefits: As you can tell from the name of this point, it is beneficial for insomnia. Use this point also for ankle pain, back pain, and hypertension.

Bladder Meridian No. 60—High Mountain

To find this point, move your finger to the outside of the ankle, between the outside ankle bone and the Achilles' tendon. Press and hold for one minute.

Additional Benefits: Press on this point for lower-back pain and rheumatism. This is an excellent pain-reliever point for the lower back.

Kidney Meridian No. 6—Illuminated Sea

This point is on the inside of the ankle, one thumb width directly below the ankle bone. Press and hold for thirty to sixty seconds.

Additional Benefits: Use this point for sore heels, swollen ankles, and ankle pain.

Gallbladder Meridian No. 40—Wilderness Mound

This pressure point is particularly effective for a sprained ankle. Find the large hollow directly below the outside ankle bone and press for up to ten minutes by alternating firm and light touches. Repeat as often as necessary until the pain begins to lessen.

Additional Benefits: This point is equally beneficial for side aches, shoulder pain, and headaches. Use this point also for a sprained ankle or the pain of sciatica.

Knee Pain

Stomach Meridian No. 35—Calf's Nose

This pressure point is located on the outside of the leg below the kneecap. If you have trouble finding the small hollow, lift your leg slightly off the floor. Press and hold with your middle finger while leaning forward from the waist to give yourself more leverage. Hold for one minute.

Additional Benefits: Use this point for swelling of the lower legs, ankles and feet, for knee pain, and rheumatism in the feet.

Bladder Meridian No. 53—Commanding Activity

Find this pressure point by tracing your finger along the crease at the back of your knee toward the outside edge. Press with your middle finger, ring, and index fingers supporting and lean forward for firmer pressure.

Additional Benefits: Use this point for problems with urination. This is also an effective point to relieve knee stiffness and pain, spasms in the calf muscles, and when you are feeling faint.

Liver Meridian No. 8—Crooked Spring

This pressure point is located along the knee crease on the inside of the knee. Press and hold with your thumb for thirty to sixty seconds.

Additional Benefits: This point is effective for regulating the menstrual cycle and for vaginal or penile pain. Use this point also for knee pain, fibroids, and to strengthen knees.

Kidney Meridian No. 10—Nourishing Valley

Find this point by tracing your finger along the crease at the back of the knee toward the inside edge. Press your thumb between the two tendons and hold for one minute.

Additional Benefits: Use this point for abdominal cramps and pain. This point is also effective to relieve knee pain and genital disorders.

Spleen Meridian No. 9—Shady Side of the Mountain

On the inside of the leg just below the bulge that is under the side of the knee is the top of the shinbone. If you have difficulty finding this point, use the pressure-points diagram at the end of this chapter. Press firmly with your middle finger and hold for thirty to sixty seconds.

Additional Benefits: This is an effective point to reduce the pain of varicose veins. Because this pressure point regulates the water pathways of the body, it is useful for reducing water retention, swelling, and edema particularly around the knee.

Gallbladder Meridian No. 34—Sunny Side of the Mountain

As the name implies this point is on the opposite side of your leg, i.e., on the outside at the head of the shinbone. Press and hold for one minute using your middle finger supported by the ring and index fingers. Lean forward for more leverage.

Additional Benefits: Use this point for the pain of sciatica as well as for knee pain. This pressure point relaxes all the muscles of the lower body and should be used if you have overused these muscles.

Cramps and Spasms

Liver Meridian No. 3—Bigger Rushing

Press your middle finger in the valley between the big toe and the second toe at its highest point. Hold for one minute.

Additional Benefits: Use this point for tired eyes and headaches. This pressure point clears and invigorates the whole system so it is effective for relieving arthritis pain, headaches, tired eyes, hangovers, and nasal congestion and pain.

Governing Vessel Meridian No. 26—Middle of a Person

This point is located directly between the base of the nose bone and the top of the ridge of the gums. Press firmly and hold for one minute.

Additional Benefits: This point is most effective for fainting and dizzy spells. Use this point also for hay fever and to clear your mind.

Bladder Meridian No. 57—Supporting Mountain

This point is at the base of the calf muscle, midway between the crease at the back of your knee and your heel. Press and hold with your thumb for one minute.

Additional Benefits: Use this point to relieve stomachaches and leg pain and to reduce swelling of the legs. This point is also effective for strengthening the lower back.

Diarrhea

Spleen Meridian No. 16—Abdominal Sorrow

Trace along the bottom of your rib cage from the outside edge to ½ inch inward from the nipple line. Press on this point with your middle finger and hold for thirty to sixty seconds.

Additional Benefits: This point may also be used for nausea, abdominal cramps and ulcer pain. Because this pressure point balances the appetite and gastrointestinal system, use this point if you are trying to lose weight.

Spleen Meridian No. 4—Grandfather Grandson

From the sole of your foot, measure one thumb width toward the arch. To make it easier to press firmly on this point, rest your ankle on the knee of your other leg and hold for one minute.

Additional Benefits: Use for menstrual cramps as well as diarrhea. This is an effective point to use regularly in order to stabilize and strengthen your digestive system.

Conception Vessel Meridian No. 6—Sea of Energy

To find this point, measure two finger widths below your navel. Press strongly and hold for at least one minute.

Additional Benefits: This point may also be used for constipation. This is an effective point for strengthening the lower back and to replenish your reserves of energy.

Liver Meridian No. 2—Travel Between

Press on the junction of skin between the big toe and the second toe. Hold for one minute.

Additional Benefits: This point is effective for calming the spirit. Use this point for diarrhea as well as stomachaches and nausea.

Menstrual Cramps and Bloating

Conception Vessel No. 4—Gate Origin

Measure four finger widths below the navel. Press firmly and hold for one minute.

Additional Benefits: This is an effective pressure point for incontinence. Use this point for impotence and insomnia.

Spleen Meridian No. 12—Rushing Door
Spleen Meridian No. 13—Mansion Cottage

These two points are located in the pelvic area in the middle of the creases where the legs are joined to the trunk. Press and hold with your middle finger for one minute.

Additional Benefits: Use this point for the relief of abdominal cramps and bloating. This is another effective point for impotence and menstrual cramps.

Bladder Meridian Nos. 27–34—Sacral Points

Lie on your back with one hand over the other underneath the base of the spine. Breathe deeply, in through your nose and out through your mouth, expanding and contracting your diaphragm. Hold your position for at least two minutes.

Additional Benefits: These points are beneficial for the relief of lumbago and sciatica. Use these points to relieve labor pain and for any problems of the reproductive system.

Spleen Meridian No. 6—Three Yin Crossing

Measure four finger widths upward from the ankle bone to the back of your shinbone. Slide your finger along the shinbone to the back. Press and hold for at least one minute.

Additional Benefits: Use this point for diarrhea, water retention, diabetes, and to regulate menstruation. Do not press on this point during the last two months of pregnancy.

Bladder Meridian No. 48—Womb and Vitals

The sacrum is the large bony area at the base of the spine. Midway between the top of the hip bone and the bottom of the buttocks, measure one to two finger widths to the side of the sacrum. To allow for firmer pressure, sit in a chair with a solid back, fist your hands, and lean back into your fists. Hold for at least one minute, breathing deeply while pressing against this point.

Additional Benefits: This is a very effective point to relieve the pain of sciatica and lower backache. Use this point for hip pain or muscle tension in the hip or lower back area.

Sciatica and Lower Backaches

Bladder Meridian No. 54—Commanding Middle

This point is located in the middle of the crease at the back of the knee. Press firmly with your thumbs and lead over to provide more leverage. Hold for one minute. Repeat as necessary.

Additional Benefits: Use this pressure point for knee stiffness and pain. This point strengthens the lower back and knees.

Conception Vessel Meridian No. 6—Sea of Energy

Measure two finger widths below your navel. Press firmly and deeply. Hold for at least one minute.

Additional Benefits: This is an effective point to relieve bloating, gas, and constipation. Use this point if you lower back muscles are weak or if you are feeling fatigued.

Bladder Meridians Nos. 23 and 47—Sea of Vitality

These points are located at two and four finger widths from the spine at waist level. Press strongly unless that area is tender to the touch. For a firmer pressure, sit in a solid-back chair, fist your hands, and lean into your fists. Hold for at least one minute.

Additional Benefits: Use this point to strengthen your digestive organs and kidneys. This pressure point strengthens the digestive organs, the kidneys, and the immune system.

Swelling and Water Retention

Kidney Meridian No. 2—Blazing Valley

Trace your finger along a line from the outer edge of the big toe to the middle of your arch. Press firmly and hold for at least one minute.

Additional Benefits: This pressure point is an effective remedy for irregular menstruation and is beneficial for the kidneys. Use this point also for swelling and foot cramps.

Kidney Meridian No. 6—Illuminated Sea

Measure one thumb width below the inside ankle bone. Rest your ankle on the knee of your other leg for better leverage. Press and hold for at least one minute.

Additional Benefits: Use this point to reduce ankle and heel pain.

Spleen Meridian No. 9—Shady Side of the Mountain

This point is located on the inside of the leg below the knee at the base of the kneebone. Press and hold for one minute.

Additional Benefits: This point is beneficial for releasing leg tension from overused muscles and to relieve the pain of varicose veins. Use this point also for edema and knee problems with swelling and pain.

Spleen Meridian No. 6—Three Yin Crossing

Locate your shin bone and then measure four finger widths up from your inside ankle bone at the back of your shin bone. Press and hold for at least one minute. If your leg is painful, press this point gently and hold for two minutes. Do not use this point during the last two months of pregnancy.

Additional Benefits: Use this pressure point to relieve menstrual cramps. This point is also effective for diarrhea and diabetes.

Relaxation Points

A student of mine from the local senior center is one of those people who is busier in retirement than she was while pursuing a career and raising a family. Between keeping house, baking, baby-sitting for grandchildren, out-of-state trips, and volunteer work, she is often too exhausted to fall asleep at night. Since joining the seated T'ai Chi class, she has learned about the use of pressure points. Whenever she experiences a bout of insomnia, she uses the Third Eye Point and the Wind Mansion point. With one minute of pressure on each of these points, along with deep breathing and mind-clearing visualization, she is soon fast asleep.

If stress is at the root of most illnesses then the daily practice of relaxation techniques is the key to good health. The acupressure points described in this section address three problems that may be the cause of, or symptomatic of, the stress in your daily life: depression and emotional imbalance, insomnia, and shoulder tension. Depression or emotional highs and lows may be directly related to your diet, to hormonal changes such as PMS, or to grief due to the loss of a loved one. Questions about your diet may be best directed toward your doctor or a dietitian. Consult your physician for advice and help with hormonal changes. Friends and/or a qualified counselor can be of great assistance when dealing with grief.

Insomnia is often caused by stress at home or work. Deep breathing and relaxation pressure points will relieve your mind of worries. Using the insomnia acupressure points just before bedtime will help you to fall asleep and ensure a full night's rest regardless of the cause of your sleeplessness.

Certain parts of the body are considered by Chinese health practitioners to be the collecting points for all disruptions of the body, mind, or spirit. Tension and pain in the shoulders is an indication of overall physical and/or emotional imbalance. By spending a few minutes each day, preferably morning and evening, practicing deep diaphragmatic breathing along with the shoulder healing points described here you will rebalance your entire system and enhance your feeling of general well-being.

Depression and Emotional Imbalance

Governing Vessel Meridian No. 19—Posterior Summit
Governing Vessel Meridian No. 20—One Hundred Meeting Point
Governing Vessel Meridian No. 21—Anterior Summit

First locate the point on your head where a baby's soft spot is. Press the middle finger of your right hand on this point (One Hundred Meeting Point). With your index finger, find the indentation about one finger width below this point (Posterior Summit). At about the same distance from your middle finger toward the front of your head is the Anterior Summit. Use your ring finger to press on this point. All three fingers should be exerting the same pressure at the same time. Hold for at least one minute.

Additional Benefits: Use these three points in the same way for headaches and vertigo. These three pressure points also clear the brain and calm the spirit.

Kidney Meridian No. 27—Elegant Mansion

This point is located between the collarbone and the first rib alongside the breastbone. Press firmly and hold for one minute.

Additional Benefits: This is a highly effective point to reduce the breathing difficulties of asthma and to relieve a sore throat. This point generally benefits the lungs, throat, and kidneys.

Gallbladder Meridian No. 20—Gates of Consciousness

There are two sets of muscles in the neck that are easy to feel with your fingers. The larger ropy set of muscles closest to the spine are the trapezius muscles. Another set of neck muscles one to two finger widths to the side of each of the trapezius muscles is the sternoclineidomastoid muscles that connect to the mastoid bones behind the ears. Trace outward at the base of the skull on either side of your spine until you find the two large sets of muscles in your neck. Press firmly between these two sets of muscles and hold for one minute.

Additional Benefits: Use this point for dizziness and headaches. This is also an effective point to relieve neck and stiffness, insomnia, and hypertension.

Bladder Meridian No. 10—Heavenly Pillar

Half an inch below the base of the skull, in the middle of the large neck muscle (trapezius) closest to the spine is the point called Heavenly Pillar. Press firmly on this point for one minute.

Additional Benefits: This point is beneficial for the relief of insomnia and physical or mental overexertion. Use this point also for stress, burnout, and overexertion.

Lung Meridian No. 1—Letting Go

Measure four finger widths from the upper end of the armpit crease and one finger width inward toward the middle of the chest. Press and hold for thirty to sixty seconds.

Additional Benefits: Use this point for relief of a cough or asthma. This pressure point also clears the chest of congestion and strengthens the lungs while it reduces fatigue.

Conception Vessel Meridian No. 17—Sea of Tranquillity

Find the base of your breastbone and measure three finger widths upward. Press and hold for one minute.

Additional Benefits: This is an effective point for chest congestion due to colds or the flu. This pressure point also balances the emotions and calms the spirit so you can use this point everyday to keep yourself on an even keel.

Governing Vessel Meridian No. 24.5—Third Eye Point

The Third Eye Point is located between your eyebrows and above the nose bone in a small indentation. Press with one finger or steeple your hands and press with both index fingers. Hold for at least one minute.

Additional Benefits: Use this point to increase your intuitive and creative abilities. This pressure point balances all the glands, stimulates the activities of the immune system, and calms the spirit as well.

Insomnia

Pericardium Meridian No. 6—Inner Gate

Measure two and a half finger widths upward on your arm from the wrist crease. In the middle of your forearm, press and hold for one minute. Repeat as necessary. Close your eyes and breathe deeply as you hold this point.

Additional Benefits: This point is beneficial to relieve indigestion and nausea. Use this point also to relieve wrist pain and sleeplessness.

Heart Meridian No. 7—Spirit Gate

This point is located at the end of the wrist crease directly below your little finger. Press and hold for thirty to sixty seconds while you breathe deeply and relax.

Additional Benefits: Use this point to strengthen your heart muscle and relieve feelings of anxiety. This pressure point also regulates the heart and strengthens the spirit.

Governing Vessel Meridian No. 24.5—Third Eye Point

Steeple your fingers and press both index fingers on the small indentation between your eyebrows at the top of the nose bone. Close your eyes and hold for at least one minute while breathing deeply.

Additional Benefits: This pressure point rebalances all the glands. Use this point also to clear your mind and stimulate creativity.

Governing Vessel Meridian No. 16—Wind Mansion

There is a large hollow at the back of the end below the base of the skull. Press firmly and hold for one minute.

Additional Benefits: Use this point to clear sinus cavities and nasal passages. This point is also effective for neck aches, headaches, nose bleeds, and sore throats.

Shoulder Tension and Pain

Gallbladder Meridian No. 20—Gates of Consciousness

Find the two large vertical neck muscles on either side of your spine (the trapezius and the sternoclineidomastoid). Press your middle fingers on each side of your spine below the base of the neck in between these two sets of muscles. Press deeply and hold for one minute.

Additional Benefits: This is an effective point for the relief of headaches. Use this point for relieving a stiff neck, insomnia, and hypertension.

Triple Warmer Meridian No. 15—Heavenly Rejuvenation

There is a large muscle at the top of your shoulders. Press with your middle fingers 1/2 inch below that muscle midway between the base of the neck and the outside of the shoulders. Hold for one minute.

Additional Benefits: Use this pressure point to increase your immunity to colds. This is also an effective point to relax your shoulders and alleviate shoulder pain.

Large Intestine Meridian No. 14—Outer Arm Bone

Trace the large bone on the outside of your arm approximately one-third of the way between the shoulder and the elbow. Press on the muscle at this point and hold for at least one minute.

Additional Benefits: This point is also beneficial for the relief of toothaches. Use this point also to reduce aching in the arms and for a stiff neck.

Gallbladder Meridian No. 21—Shoulder Well

Approximately 1 to 2 inches from the base of the neck at the top of the shoulder is the Shoulder Well. Press firmly on this point with your opposite hand, i.e., use your right middle finger on your left shoulder and vice versa. Hold for one minute then change sides.

Additional Benefits: Use this point to reduce feelings of irritability. This point softens hard or tense muscles and is effective for reducing general fatigue.

A Final Word

T'ai Chi is not a quick fix. It was intended from its inception to be the subject of life-long practice. The one virtue that is required in the practice of T'ai Chi is patience—patience with yourself and patience with the process of the art itself. In the Orient, breathing techniques, herbal medicine, acupuncture, and the like were not developed to be used for a short time and then discarded. They are designed to promote well-being, cure ills, and slow down the aging process over a period of years, not months. We in the United States have been led to expect an instantaneous cure for everything from the common cold to chronic diseases. Yet, common sense tells us that this is not possible. Perhaps that is why we are so dissatisfied with our medical practitioners and why we so overuse drugs.

Aging is a slow and inevitable process and chronic disease does not appear overnight. We must be willing to invest the necessary time and effort to achieve a cure and renew at least some of our youthful vigor. Although you may be learning T'ai Chi for the first time as a mature adult, you will benefit from it if you are faithful and disciplined in its use. The Three Treasures that the Chinese found and identified thousands of years ago are no less precious today. Whether you choose to use the full fifty minutes of the T'ai Chi exercises or the fifteen-minute sets described in Chapter 4, I believe you will find, as I did, that you will be more physically fit, your mind will be clearer, and your spirit calmer no matter what pressures you face each day. It is my hope that you will find these exercises so enjoyable and refreshing that you will look forward each day to the time you've set aside for your practice.

Appendix A

Meridian Abbreviations

The following is a list of the abbreviations used in acupressure and acupuncture to identify the trigger points on the body. The letters indicate the meridian on which each point is located.

Lu	Lung
LI	Large Intestine
Sp	Spleen
TW	Triple Warmer
St	Stomach
SI	Small Intestine
H	Heart
CV	Conception Vessel
K	Kidney
P	Pericardium
B	Bladder
GB	Gallbladder
Lv	Liver
GV	Governing Vessel

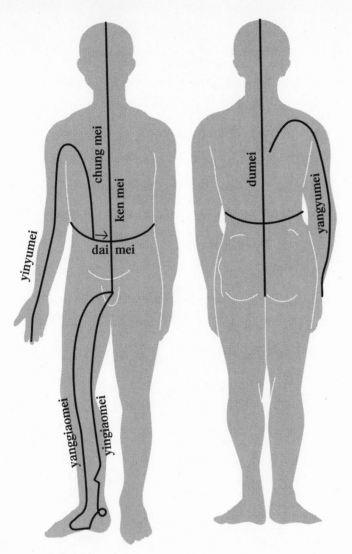

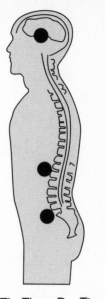

The Three Dan Tiens

Beginnings Chart

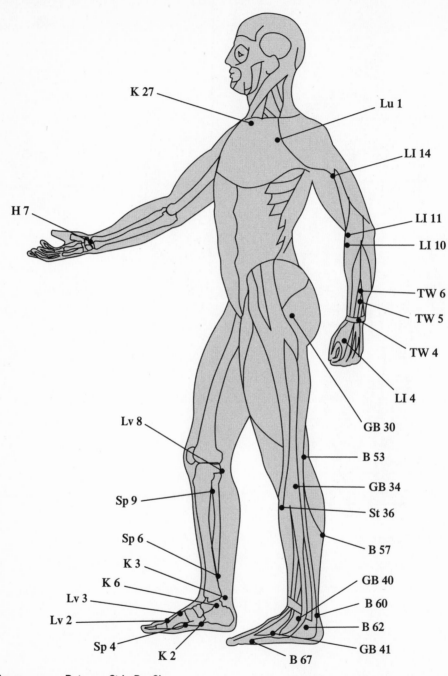

K 27

Lu 1

LI 14

H 7

LI 11

LI 10

TW 6

TW 5

TW 4

LI 4

GB 30

Lv 8

B 53

GB 34

Sp 9

St 36

B 57

Sp 6

K 3

GB 40

K 6

B 60

Lv 3

B 62

Lv 2

Sp 4

GB 41

K 2

B 67

Acupressure Points—Side Profile

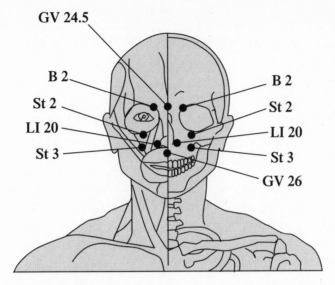

Acupressure Points—Head Frontal

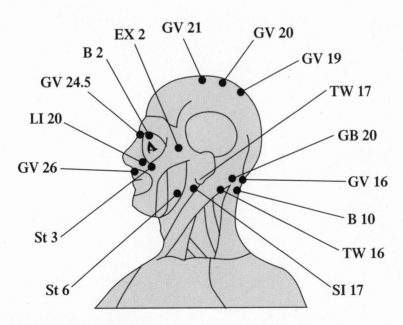

Acupressure Points—Head Profile

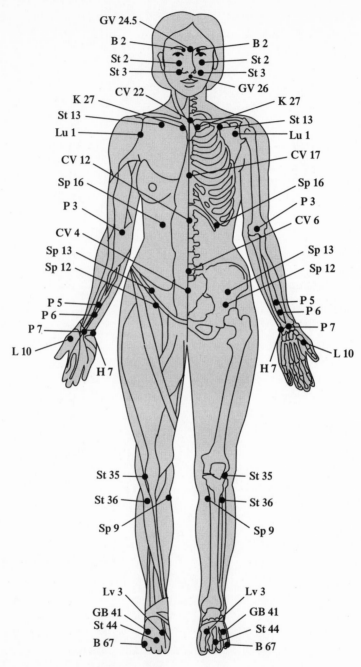

GV 24.5
B 2
St 2
St 3
CV 22
K 27
St 13
Lu 1
CV 12
Sp 16
P 3
CV 4
Sp 13
Sp 12
P 5
P 6
P 7
L 10
H 7
B 2
St 2
St 3
GV 26
K 27
St 13
Lu 1
CV 17
Sp 16
P 3
CV 6
Sp 13
Sp 12
P 5
P 6
P 7
L 10
H 7
St 35
St 36
Sp 9
St 35
St 36
Sp 9
Lv 3
GB 41
St 44
B 67
Lv 3
GB 41
St 44
B 67

Acupressure Points—Female Figure Front

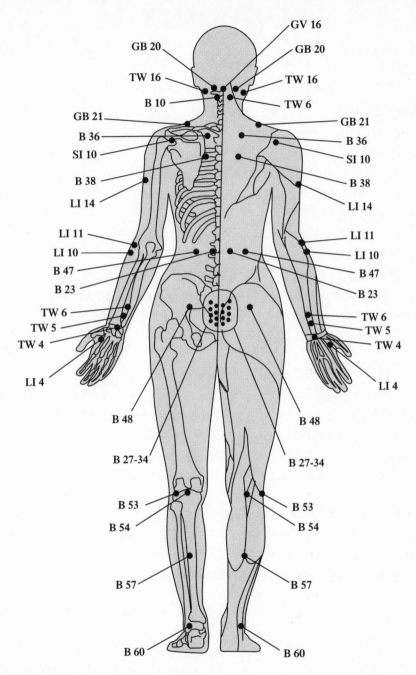

GV 16
GB 20
GB 20
TW 16
TW 16
TW 6
B 10
GB 21
GB 21
B 36
B 36
SI 10
SI 10
B 38
B 38
LI 14
LI 14
LI 11
LI 11
LI 10
LI 10
B 47
B 47
B 23
B 23
TW 6
TW 6
TW 5
TW 5
TW 4
TW 4
LI 4
LI 4
B 48
B 48
B 27-34
B 27-34
B 53
B 53
B 54
B 54
B 57
B 57
B 60
B 60

Acupressure Points—Female Figure Back

Appendix A

Appendix B

Suggested Readings

Chuckrow, Robert (1998). *The Tai Chi Book*, Boston, MA. YMAA Publication Center.

Crompton, Paul (1987). *The T'ai Chi Workbook*, Boston, MA. Shambala.

Dalton, Jerry O. (1994). *Backward Down the Path*, New York, NY Avon Books.

Gach, Michael Reed (1990). *Acupressure's Potent Points*, New York, NY. Bantam Books.

Ming-Dao, Deng (1992). *365 Tao*, New York, NY. Harper San Francisco.

Schorre, Jane (1997). *How to Grasp the Bird's Tail If You Don't Speak Chinese*, Houston, TX. Arts of China Seminars.

Recommended Music

The following music titles are available through Wayfarer Publications. To write and request a catalog or any of the music listed, address your request to Wayfarer Publications, P.O. Box 39938, Los Angeles, California 90039. If you would prefer to call for the catalog or an order, the number is (323) 665-7773; for credit-card purchases only, call toll free,1-800-888-9119.

Qigong Melody, CD 6123; Tape 6124
Music for Calming Emotions, CD 6137; Tape 6138
Music for Invigorating the Spirit, CD 6139; Tape 6140
Return to Simplicity, CD 6215; Tape 6216
Tranquility, CD 6213; Tape 6214

Bibliography

Bankart, C. Peter (1997). *Talking Cures*, Pacific Grove, CA. Brooks/Cole Publishing Company.

Beling, Janna (1999). 'Twelve month Tai Chi training in the elderly: its effects on health fitness." *Physical Therapy*, v.79 i2, p. 208 (1).

Birdsall, George (1997). *The Feng Shui Companion*, Rochester, VT. Destiny Books.

Capra, Fritjof (1991). *The Tao of Physics*, Boston, MA. Shambala.

Capra, Fritjof (1983). *The Turning Point*, New York, NY. Bantam Books.

Cerrato, Paul L. (1999). "Tai Chi: a martial art turns therapeutic." RN, v.62 i2, p.59(2).

Chuckrow, Robert (1998). *The Tai Chi Book*, Boston, MA. YMAA Publication Center.

Crompton, Paul (1987). *The T'ai Chi Workbook*, Boston, MA. Shambala

Dalton, Jerry O. (1994). *Backward Down the Path*, New York, NY. Avon Books

Gach, Michael Reed (1990). *Acupressure's Potent Points*, New York, NY. Bantam Books.

Kessenich, Cathy R. (1998). "Tai Chi as a method of fall prevention in the elderly." *Orthopaedic Nursing*, July—August, v.17 n4, p.27(3).

Lewis, Dennis (1997). *The Tao of Natural Breathing*, San Francisco, CA. Mountain Wind Publishing.

Liao, Waysun (1995). *The Essence of T'ai Chi*, Boston, MA. Shambala.

LoBuono, Charlotte and Pinkowish, Mary (1999). "Moderate exercise, Tai Chi improves blood pressure in older adults." *Patient Care*, v.33 i18, p.230.

Ming-Dao, Deng (1992). *365 Tao*, New York, NY. Harper San Francisco.

Schorre, Jane (1997). *How to Grasp the Bird's Tail If You Don't Speak Chinese*, Houston, TX. Arts of China Seminars.

Wing, R. L. (1986). *The Tao of Power*, New York, NY. Doubleday.